THE USE OF THE SELF

By Wilfred Barlow

The Alexander Principle

THE USE OF THE SELF

Its Conscious Direction in Relation to Diagnosis
Functioning and the Control of Reaction

by

F. MATTHIAS ALEXANDER

With an Introduction by Wilfred Barlow

*Dedicated to all those who by their
interest and participation in my work
have helped me to gain the experience
set down in this book*

An Orion paperback

First published in Great Britain in 1932
by Methuen & Co. Ltd
This paperback edition published in 1985
by Victor Gollancz

Reissued 2001
by Orion Books Ltd,
Orion House, 5 Upper St Martin's Lane,
London WC2H 9EA

An Hachette UK company

11

A CIP catalogue record for this book is available
from the British Library.

ISBN 978-0-7528-4391-9

Printed and bound in Great Britain by
Clays Ltd, St Ives plc

The Orion Publishing Group's policy is to use papers that
are natural, renewable and recyclable products and
made from wood grown in sustainable forests. The logging
and manufacturing processes are expected to conform to
the environmental regulations of the country of origin.

www.orionbooks.co.uk

CONTENTS

INTRODUCTION TO THE 1985 EDITION

by Wilfred Barlow

When *The Use of the Self* was first published in 1932 the *British Medical Journal* called it a classic — a classic of scientific observation. With this reissue in 1985, it has become a different sort of classic: one of the few books which simply will not die. Persistent demand has kept it alive.

It is not a classic piece of literature. Alexander's prose-style did not come easily to him, and many of us sat at his side whilst he attemped to get more and more information into sentences which became longer and longer, more and more ponderous. Its classic nature lies in a content which is as novel today as it was fifty years ago.

Alexander died in 1955, about twenty years before his 'Alexander Principle'* was to receive world-wide recognition. There had, of course, been many forms of recognition in his life-time. John Dewey's writings — and especially the admirable introductions to Alexander's books — placed his work fairly and squarely above the level of some manipulative therapy or relaxation technique: the pigeon-holes into which many people had tried to put him.

The essentially philosophical nature of his work was not at first easily recognized. Low's cartoon, printed in the original edition, shows an academic, surrounded by books, looking at himself in a mirror, with a caption which reads 'The little thing which puzzles him is himself'. Alexander's work was and is concerned with the intimate management of our moment-to-moment perceptions of ourselves.

The Alexander Principle, Wilfred Barlow. Gollancz, 1973.

In *The Use of the Self* we find not only a very special type of
self-observation, but also the willingness to question our
preconceptions, and to realize that what seemed right yester-
day might not be right today. When Nikolaas Tinbergen gave
his Nobel oration in 1973,* he stressed the importance of
observation, of 'watching and wondering'. He devoted half of
his oration to Alexander's observation of human beings ' . . .
this basic scientific method is still too often looked down on by
those blinded by the glamour of apparatus. A little more
attention to the body as a whole and to the unity of body and
mind could substantially expand the field of medical research.'

What was it that Alexander observed, and in what way was
his method of observation so novel? First of all he observed
that the *use* of the head/neck region was of paramount
importance for psycho-physical functioning. The first chapter
of this book details his painstaking observation — an observation which was to be resoundingly endorsed by a recent
symposium on his work at the University of New South Wales
in his native Sydney: a symposium which brought together
scientists from all over the world, and which was to indicate
how Alexander, in his work on awareness of the head/neck
region, had preceded by nearly a hundred years the most
up-to-date findings on *Proprioception, Posture, and Emotion* (the title of the symposium).†

Not only did Alexander delineate the nature of bodily misuse, but, more importantly, he devised a method of extreme
subtlety by means of which we can re-educate our faulty
habits. The importance of Alexander's way of 'ordering' of the
body will become clearer as more and more people apply
themselves to it.

The trickle of interest in Alexander's method has now
become a torrent. It has become a torrent because it works,

---

*'Ethology and Stress diseases'. Nikolaas Tinbergen in *More Talk of
Alexander*. Gollancz, 1979.

†*Proprioception, Posture, and Emotion*, ed. David Garlick. The Commit-
tee in Postgraduate Medical Education. The University of New South Wales,
1982.

and at last it is sweeping away much of the rubbish which has cluttered up progress in this field. We can only marvel at the courage, clear-sightedness and perseverance which underlies this book.

1985   W.B.

INTRODUCTION

by Professor John Dewey

Reprinted from the 1939 edition

In writing some introductory words to Mr Alexander's previous book, *Constructive Conscious Control of the Individual*, I stated that his procedure and conclusions meet all the requirements of the strictest scientific method, and that he has applied the method in a field in which it had never been used before — that of our judgments and beliefs concerning ourselves and our activities. In so doing, he has, I said in effect, rounded out the results of the sciences in the physical field, accomplishing this end in such a way that they become capable of use for human benefit. It is a commonplace that scientific technique has for its consequence control of the energies to which it refers. Physical science has for its fruit an astounding degree of new command of physical energies. Yet we are faced with a situation which is serious, perhaps tragically so. There is everywhere increasing doubt as to whether this physical mastery of physical energies is going to further human welfare, or whether human happiness is going to be wrecked by it. Ultimately there is but one sure way of answering this question in the hopeful and constructive sense. If there can be developed a technique which will enable individuals really to secure the right use of themselves, then the factor on which depends the final use of all other forms of energy will be brought under control. Mr Alexander has evolved this technique.

In repeating these statements, I do so fully aware of

their sweeping nature. Were not our eyes and ears so accustomed to irresponsible statements that we cease to ask for either meaning or proof, they might well raise a question as to the complete intellectual responsibility and competency of their author. In repeating them after the lapse of intervening years, I appeal to the account which Mr Alexander has given of the origin of his discovery of the principle of central and conscious control. Those who do not identify science with a parade of technical vocabulary will find in this account the essentials of scientific method in any field of inquiry. They will find a record of long-continued, patient, unwearied experimentation and observation in which every inference is extended, tested, corrected by further more searching experiments; they will find a series of such observations in which the mind is carried from observation of comparatively coarse, gross, superficial connections of causes and effect to those causal conditions which are fundamental and central in the use which we make of ourselves.

Personally, I cannot speak with too much admiration — in the original sense of wonder as well as the sense of respect — of the persistence and thoroughness with which these extremely difficult observations and experiments were carried out. In consequence, Mr Alexander created what may be truly called a physiology of the *living* organism. His observations and experiments have to do with the actual functioning of the body, with the organism in operation, and in operation under the ordinary conditions of living — rising, sitting, walking, standing, using arms, hands, voice, tools, instruments of all kinds. The contrast between sustained and accurate observations of the living and the usual activities of man and those made upon dead things under unusual and artificial conditions marks the difference between true and pseudo-science. And yet so used have we become to associating 'science' with the latter sort of thing that its contrast with the genuinely scientific character of Mr Alexander's observations has been one great reason for the failure of many to appreciate his technique and conclusions.

As might be anticipated, the conclusions of Mr Alexander's experimental inquiries are in harmony with what physiologists know about the muscular and nervous structure. But they give a new significance to that knowledge; indeed, they make evident what knowledge itself really is. The anatomist may 'know' the exact function of each muscle, and conversely know what muscles come into play in the execution of any specified act. But if he is himself unable to co-ordinate all the muscular structures involved in, say, sitting down or in rising from a sitting position in a way which achieves the optimum and efficient performance of that act — if, in other words, he misuses himself in what he does — how can he be said to *know* in the full and vital sense of that word? Magnus proved by means of what may be called *external* evidence the existence of a central control in the organism. But Mr Alexander's technique gave a direct and intimate confirmation in personal experience of the fact of central control long before Magnus carried on his investigations. And one who has had experience of the technique *knows* it through the series of experiences which he himself has. The genuinely scientific character of Mr Alexander's teaching and discoveries can be safely rested upon this fact alone.

The vitality of a scientific discovery is revealed and tested in its power to project and direct new further operations which not only harmonize with prior results, but which lead on to new observed materials, suggesting in turn further experimentally controlled acts, and so on in a continued series of new developments. Speaking as a pupil, it was because of this fact as demonstrated in personal experience that I first became convinced of the scientific quality of Mr Alexander's work. Each lesson was a laboratory experimental demonstration. Statements made in advance of consequences to follow and the means by which they would be reached were met with implicit scepticism — a fact which is practically inevitable, since, as Mr Alexander points out, one uses the very conditions that need re-education as one's standard of judgment. Each lesson carries the process somewhat farther and confirms in the most intimate and convincing fashion the claims that are made. As one goes on, new areas are opened, new possibilities are seen and then realized; one finds himself continually growing, and realizes that there is an endless process of growth initiated.

From one standpoint, I had an unusual opportunity for making an intellectual study of the technique and its results. I was, from the practical standpoint, an inept, awkward, and slow pupil. There were no speedy and seemingly miraculous changes to evoke gratitude emotionally, while they misled me intellectually. I was forced to observe carefully at every step of the process, and to interest myself in the theory of the operations. I did this partly from my previous interest in psychology and philosophy, and partly as a compensation for my practical backwardness. In bringing to bear whatever knowledge I already possessed — or thought I did — and whatever powers of discipline in mental application I had acquired in the pursuit of these studies, I had the most humiliating experience of my life, intellectually speaking. For to find that one is unable to execute directions, including inhibitory ones, in doing such a seemingly simple act as to sit down, when one is using all the mental capacity which one prides himself upon possessing, is not an experience congenial to one's vanity. But it may be conducive to analytic study of causal conditions, obstructive and positive. And so I verified in personal experience all that Mr Alexander says about the unity of the physical and psychical in the psycho-physical; about our habitually wrong use of ourselves; and the part this wrong use plays in generating all kinds of unnecessary tensions and wastes of energy; about the vitiation of our sensory appreciations which form the material of our judgments of ourselves; about the unconditional necessity of inhibition of customary acts, and the tremendous mental difficulty found in not 'doing' something as soon as an habitual act is suggested, together with the great change in moral and mental attitude that takes place as proper co-ordinations are established. In re-affirming my conviction as to the scientific character of Mr Alexander's discoveries and technique, I do so then not as one who has experienced a 'cure,' but as one who has brought whatever intellectual capacity he has to the study of a problem. In the study I found the things which I had 'known' — in the sense of theoretical belief — in philosophy and psychology, changed into vital experiences which gave a new meaning to knowledge of them.

In the present state of the world it is evident that the control we have gained of physical energies, heat, light, electricity, etc, without having first secured control of our use of ourselves is a perilous affair. Without control of our use of ourselves, our use of other things is blind; it may lead to anything.

Moreover, if our habitual judgments of ourselves are warped because they are based on vitiated sense material — as they must be if our habits of managing ourselves are already wrong — then the more complex the social conditions under which we live, the more disastrous must be the outcome. Every additional complication of outward instrumentalities is likely to be a step nearer destruction: a fact which the present state of the world tragically exemplifies.

The school of Pavloff has made current the idea of conditioned reflexes. Mr Alexander's work extends and corrects the idea. It proves that there are certain basic, central organic habits and attitudes which condition *every* act we perform, every use we make of ourselves. Hence a conditioned reflex is not just a matter of an arbitrarily established connection, such as that between the sound of a bell and the eating-reaction in a dog, but goes back to central conditions within the organism itself. This discovery corrects the ordinary conception of the conditioned reflex. The latter as usually understood renders an individual a passive puppet to be played upon by external manipulations. The discovery of a central control which conditions all other reactions brings the conditioning factor under conscious direction and enables the individual through his own co-ordinated activities to take possession of his own potentialities. It converts the fact of conditioned reflexes from a principle of external enslavement into a means of vital freedom.

Education is the only sure method which mankind possesses for directing his own course. But we have been involved in a vicious circle. Without knowledge of what constitutes a truly normal and healthy psycho-physical life, our professed education is likely to be mis-education. Every serious student of the formation of disposition and character which takes place in the family and school knows — speaking without the slightest exaggeration — how often and how deplorably this possibility is realized. The technique of Mr Alexander gives to the educator a standard of psycho-physical health — in which what we call morality is included. It supplies also the 'means whereby' this standard may be progressively and endlessly achieved, becoming a conscious possession of the one educated. It provides therefore the conditions for the central direction of all special educational processes. It bears the same relation to education that education itself bears to all other human activities.

I cannot therefore state too strongly the hopes that are aroused in me by the information contained in the Appendix that Mr Alexander has, with his coadjutors, opened a training class, nor my sense of the importance that this work secures adequate support. It contains in my judgment the promise and potentiality of the new direction that is needed in all education.

J. D.

PREFACE

Since the publication of my last book I have been much encouraged to receive written recognition of the value and scope of my technique from members both of the medical and educational professions, and as we are finishing the preparation of the subject matter of this book, I have received from Mr J. E. R. McDonagh, FRCS, a copy of the third volume of his book *The Nature of Disease* (Heinemann), in which he has devoted Chapter I, entitled 'Mal-co-ordination and Disease', to a review of my work. Mr McDonagh's opening lines may be of interest to the reader.

> In the epilogue to the second part of *The Nature of Disease* the author announced his intention to correlate with medicine Mr F. M. Alexander's work on the conscious control of the individual. The announcement was made because it became apparent to the author after meeting Mr Alexander and watching his technique, that the wrong use of the body plays an important role in disease. Now that the time has come to fulfil the promise the author is less sanguine of success. This is partly because Alexander's view is possibly even more fundamental than the author's view that there is only one disease, partly because the written word can neither convey the whole idea nor satisfactorily describe the technique, and partly because to link any subject with medicine it is necessary to commit the basic error of practising differentiation instead of correlation.

Other medical men are giving me their support as will be seen from what they have written in the Open Letter in the

Appendix of this present book, and I believe that in Chapter V I have indicated how medical diagnosis may be made more complete by the inclusion in medical training of the principles and procedure that I advocate.

It has been suggested to me by a friend and pupil who has read the manuscript of the first chapter of this book, that some readers may conclude from it that my technique is limited in its usefulness to dealing with serious difficulties such as those which I describe. This is not the case, however, for pupils free from any such difficulties have frequently come to me because they believed — and results justified this belief — that however well endowed they might be with health or other gifts, they would derive benefit from learning how to direct and control the use of themselves consciously in their daily activities.

Readers of my former books are aware of my special interest in the training of children, and what I have just written applies particularly to their early training. In this connexion I would refer to the benefits derived by the children and young people in our little school where they learn to put into practice the technique for the direction of an improved use of themselves in all their 'doings', in their reading, writing, etc.

I am also pleased to be able to state that the first course for the training of teachers of my work was inaugurated in March this year, and I wish to take this opportunity to thank Mr Rugg-Gunn, FRCS, for his article entitled 'A New Profession' which he recently wrote for *Women's Employment* (June, 1931), in which he pointed out the advantages for young people of taking up this work as a professional career and also referred to the work done in the little school. The publication of this article has brought so many enquiries that I have decided to include in an Appendix a reprint of the Open Letter to Intending Students of the Training Course and also a special reference to the work being done in the little school where the children are helped to put into practice the principles and procedures inherent in my technique during their school work, whatever the subject that is engaging their attention.

The results of the series of experiences I have outlined in

Chapter I seem to me to imply that in the process of acquiring a conscious direction of the use of the human organism, a hitherto 'undiscovered country' is opened up, where the scope for the development of human potentialities is practically unlimited, and anyone who chooses to take the time and trouble to carry out the procedures necessary for acquiring a conscious direction of use can put this to the test.

I would venture to suggest that even the meagre amount of knowledge of the use of the self contained in these pages may be sufficient to enable workers in all fields of investigation, whether in biology, astronomy, physics, philosophy, psychology or any other, to realize that in their researches they have passed over a field of experience which, if explored, would add new material to the premises from which to make their several deductions. After all, the self is the instrument through which all these workers must express themselves. If, therefore, a knowledge of how to direct consciously the use of the psycho-physical mechanisms of the self were made the common starting-point of their researches, this would surely tend both to unite and amplify the results of their several labours more than anything that has so far been done.

I wish to take this opportunity to thank Professor John Dewey for giving me once more his invaluable support and for allowing me to quote from his book, *Experience and Nature*. I also wish to thank Dr Peter Macdonald for reading the manuscript and for making his valuable criticisms and suggestions, and Miss Ethel Webb and Miss Irene Tasker for preparing the subject matter for publication. I am especially indebted to Miss Webb and Miss Tasker for their valuable and untiring help, without which the publication of the book would have been delayed. I am further indebted to Miss Mary Olcott and Miss Edith Lawson for their careful revision of the proofs, to Miss Evelyn Glover for her help with the final preparation of the typescript, and to two of my students, Mr George Trevelyan and Mr Gurney MacInnes, for undertaking the task of making the Index. I also desire to thank Sir Arthur Eddington for his permission to quote from his lecture on

'Science and Religion', Dr A. Murdoch for permission to quote from his Address to the St Andrew's (James Mackenzie) Institute, and Sir Edward Holderness for allowing me to quote from his article, 'The Fearful Foozler'.

24th July, 1931   F. MATTHIAS ALEXANDER

PREFACE TO NEW EDITION [1941]

The need for a new printing of this book affords me an opportunity to try to clear up certain difficulties mentioned in letters from some of my readers, difficulties which arise in trying to teach themselves to apply my technique. What troubles most of them is: 'How to do it'. Some of these correspondents have rated me quite severely because, as they put it, they are not able to teach themselves from what I have written down in my books. Yet they must be well aware that, in spite of all the textbooks on the subjects, many people are unable to teach themselves to drive a car, play golf, ski, or even to master such comparatively simple subjects as geography, history and arithmetic, without the aid of a teacher.

They should not be surprised, therefore, if they find that they are unsuccessful in learning to apply my technique, particularly since in attempting to change and improve the use of themselves they are called upon to work to a new principle, and further, that in this process they must inevitably come into contact with hitherto unknown experiences, because the carrying-out of the necessary procedures calls for a manner of use of the self that is new and unfamiliar, and when first experienced 'feels wrong'. In any attempt therefore to apply my technique to changing and improving the use of the self, it is courting failure to continue to depend upon the 'feeling' which has been the familiar guide in the old habitual 'doing' which 'felt right', but which was obviously wrong since it led us into error.

May it not be that some of those who have complained of difficulty in trying to teach themselves, may have overlooked this point, and to that extent be responsible for their own failure? And here I would like to add a word of warning to those I am trying to help, for a study of the letters in which the writers tell of experiencing difficulty in understanding, show signs of having been written after a quick reading rather than a close and careful study of the subject matter. I read recently an article suggesting that people should practise reading quickly, although the habit of too quick reading in which understanding becomes dominated by speed — that royal road to the physical and mental derangement of mankind — is an only too common failing today. This is only one example of the habit of too quick reaction to stimuli in general, and to its prevalence may be traced most of the misunderstandings, misconception and misdirection of effort manifested by the great majority of people today in conducting matters relating to the body politic.

Again, those who have written asking for help in teaching themselves are obviously almost wholly occupied with the idea of learning 'to do it right'. In reply I would refer them to the first chapter of this book, where I put down as exactly as possible what I did and (what was still more important in the end) what I did *not* do in teaching myself. If they will look at page 27, they will see that at the beginning of my experimentation I found that I must not concern myself primarily with 'doing', as I then understood 'doing', but with *preventing myself from doing* — preventing myself, that is, from giving consent to gaining an end by means of that habitual 'doing' which resulted in my repeating the wrong use of myself that I wished to change. My record shows that the further I progressed in my search for a way to free myself from the slavery to habitual reaction in 'doing' (which I had created for myself by trusting to the guidance of my unreliable sense of feeling), the more clearly I was forced to see that my only chance of freeing myself was, *as a primary step*, to refuse to give consent to my ordinary 'doing' in carrying out any procedure.

Another omission on the part of my correspondents is that nowhere in the account of their difficulties do they refer to the primary control of use. This is particularly significant, because it was my early recognition of the need for preventing what was wrong, that led me to the discovery of the primary control of my use, and I emphasized this discovery as the all-important one in my efforts to teach myself. I ask those readers therefore, who are anxious to teach themselves, to re-read this chapter, in which I give not only an account of my difficulties but also of the means whereby I freed myself from them. They will then see that the discovery of the primary control opened up a road by which I could make a safe passage from 'idealistic theory to actual practice', as long as I relied upon a conscious instead of upon an automatic sensory guidance. We cannot do this securely while relying for guidance on 'feeling' and the will-to-do motivated by instincts, many of which have outgrown their usefulness, and which are associated with untrustworthy experiences which 'feel right'.

I can assure my readers that anyone who will follow me through the experiences I have set down, especially with regard to 'non-doing', cannot fail to benefit; but I must emphasize that they will not be following me unless they recognize:

(1) that knowledge concerned with sensory experience cannot be conveyed by the written or spoken word, so that it means to the recipient what it means to the person who is trying to convey it:

(2) that they will need to depend upon new 'means — whereby' for the gaining of their ends, and that they will 'feel wrong' at first in carrying out the procedures because these will be unfamiliar:

(3) that the attempt to bring about change involving growth, development and progressive improvement in the use and functioning of the human organism, calls necessarily for the acceptance, yes, the welcoming of the unknown in sensory experience, and this 'unknown' cannot be associated with the sensory experiences that have hitherto 'felt right'.

(4) that to 'try and get it right' by direct 'doing' is to try and reproduce what is known, and cannot lead to the 'right', the as yet 'unknown'.

To anyone who accepts these points and sees the reason for keeping them in view whilst working to principle in employing the technique, I would say: 'Go ahead, but remember that time is of the essence of the contract.' It took me years to reach a point that can be reached in a few weeks with the aid of any experienced teacher.

The real solution of the problem lies in the wide acceptance of the principle of *prevention* instead of 'cure', and the realization at long last, that the most valuable knowledge we can possess is that of the use and functioning of the self, and of the means whereby the human individual may progressively raise the standard of his health and general well-being. And to those who are advocating individual right and individual endeavour in the world today, I venture to suggest that as a training for the realization of these commendable ideals, no more fundamental experience is available than that which comes to the person who, with or without a teacher, will patiently devote the time to learning to apply the technique in the act of living. The desire that mankind will come into the heritage of full individual freedom within and without the self still remains an 'idealistic theory'. Its translation into practice will call for individual freedom *in* thought and action through the development of conscious guidance and control of the self. Then and then only will the individual be liberated from the domination of instinctive habit and the slavery of the associated automatic manner of reaction.

December 19, 1941   F. MATTHIAS ALEXANDER

CHAPTER I

Evolution of a Technique

> First, then, I must request men not to suppose that . . . I wish to found
> a new sect in philosophy. For this is not what I am about; nor do I
> think that it matters much to the fortunes of men what abstract
> notions one may entertain concerning nature and the principles of
> things; and no doubt many old theories of this kind can be revived and
> many new ones introduced; just as many theories of the heavens may
> be supposed, which agree well enough with the phenomena and yet
> differ with each other.
>
> But for my part I do not trouble myself with any such speculative
> and withal unprofitable matters. My purpose, on the contrary, is to
> try whether I cannot in very fact lay more firmly the foundations, and
> extend more widely the limits of the power and greatness of man.
>
> FRANCIS BACON (*Novum Organum* — CXVI)

My two earlier books, *Man's Supreme Inheritance* and
Constructive Conscious Control of the Individual, contain a
statement of the technique which I gradually evolved over a
period of years in my search for a means whereby faulty
conditions of use in the human organism could be improved. I
must admit that when I began my investigation, I, in common
with most people, conceived of 'body' and 'mind' as separate
parts of the same organism, and consequently believed that
human ills, difficulties and shortcomings could be classified as
either 'mental' or 'physical' and dealt with on specifically
'mental' or specifically 'physical' lines. My practical experiences, however, led me to abandon this point of view and readers
of my books will be aware that the technique described in them
is based on the opposite conception, namely, that it is
impossible to separate 'mental' and 'physical' processes in any
form of human activity.

This change in my conception of the human organism has not come about as the outcome of mere theorizing on my part. It has been forced upon me by the experiences which I have gained through my investigations in a new field of practical experimentation upon the living human being.

The letters I receive from my readers shew that a large majority of those who accept the theory of the unity of mental and physical processes in human activity, find difficulty in understanding what the practical working of this theory of unity implies. This difficulty is always coming up in my teaching, but it is possible during a course of lessons to demonstrate to the pupil how the mental and physical work together in the use of the self* in all activity. Repeated demonstration of this kind brings conviction, but since the number of pupils one can take, even in a large teaching practice, is naturally limited, the opportunities for giving this demonstration are comparatively few, and I have therefore decided in this book to start at the beginning and relate the history of the investigations which gradually led to the evolution of my technique. I shall give as fully as possible the actual details of the experiments I made, telling what I observed and experienced during the process, as I believe that by so doing I shall be giving my readers the opportunity to see for themselves the train of events which finally convinced me

(1) that the so-called 'mental' and 'physical' are not separate entities;

(2) that for this reason human ills and shortcomings cannot be classified as 'mental' or 'physical' and dealt with specifically as such, but that all training, whether it be educative or otherwise, ie, whether its object be the

---

*I wish to make it clear that when I employ the word 'use', it is not in that limited sense of the use of any specific part, as, for instance, when we speak of the use of an arm or the use of a leg, but in a much wider and more comprehensive sense applying to the working of the organism in general. For I recognize that the use of any specific part such as the arm or leg involves of necessity bringing into action the different psycho-physical mechanisms of the organism, this concerted activity bringing about the use of the specific part.

prevention* or elimination of defect, error or disease, must be based upon the indivisible unity of the human organism.

If any reader doubts this, I would ask him if he can furnish any proof that the process involved in the act, say, of lifting an arm, or of walking, talking, going to sleep, starting out to learn something, thinking out a problem, making a decision, giving or withholding consent to a request or wish, or of satisfying a need or sudden impulse, is purely 'mental' or purely 'physical'. This question raises a great many points, and I suggest that a lead may be given towards meeting them if the reader will follow me through the experiences which I will now relate.

From my early youth I took a delight in poetry and it was one of my chief pleasures to study the plays of Shakespeare, reading them aloud and endeavouring to interpret the characters. This led to my becoming interested in elocution and the art of reciting, and now and again I was asked to recite in public. I was sufficiently successful to think of taking up Shakespearean reciting as a career, and worked long and hard at the study of every branch of dramatic expression. After a certain amount of experience as an amateur, I reached the stage when I believed that my work could stand the severer test of being judged from the professional standard, and the

---

*I use the word 'prevention' (and this applies equally to 'cure') not because I consider it adequate or wholly suitable for my purpose, but because I cannot find another to take its place. 'Prevention' in its fullest sense implies the existence of satisfactory conditions which can be prevented from changing for the worse. In this sense prevention is not possible in practice today, since the conditions now present in the civilized human creature are such that it would be difficult to find anyone who is entirely free from manifestations of wrong use and functioning. When, therefore, I use the terms 'prevention' and 'cure', I use them in a relative sense only, including under 'preventive' measures all attempts to prevent faulty use and functioning of the organism generally as a means of preventing defect, disorder and disease, and under 'curative' measures those methods in which the influence of faulty use upon functioning is ignored when dealing with defects, disorder and disease.

criticisms I received justified me in deciding to take up reciting as a profession.

All went well for some years, when I began to have trouble with my throat and vocal cords, and not long after I was told by my friends that when I was reciting my breathing was audible, and that they could hear me (as they put it) 'gasping' and 'sucking in air' through my mouth. This worried me even more than my actual throat trouble which was then in its early stages, for I had always prided myself on being free from the habit of audibly sucking in breath which is so common with reciters, actors and singers. I therefore sought the advice of doctors and voice trainers in the hope of remedying my faulty breathing and relieving my hoarseness, but in spite of all that they could do in the way of treatment, the gasping and sucking in of breath when I was reciting became more and more exaggerated and the hoarseness recurred at shorter intervals.*
The treatment I was receiving became less and less effective as time went on, and the trouble gradually increased until, after a few years, I found to my dismay that I had developed a condition of hoarseness which from time to time culminated in a complete loss of voice. I had experienced a good deal of ill-health all my life and this had often been a stumbling-block to me, so that with the additional burden of my recurring hoarseness, I began to doubt the soundness of my vocal organs. The climax came when I was offered a particularly attractive and important engagement, for by this time I had reached such a stage of uncertainty about the conditions of my vocal organs that I was frankly afraid to accept it. I decided to consult my doctor once more, even though the previous treatment had been disappointing. After making a fresh

*The medical diagnosis in my case was irritation of the mucous membrane of the throat and nose, and inflammation of the vocal cords which were said to be unduly relaxed. My uvula was very long and at times caused acute attacks of coughing. For this reason two of my medical advisers recommended it should be shortened by a minor operation, but I did not follow this advice. I now have little doubt that I was suffering from what is sometimes called 'clergyman's sore throat'.

examination of my throat, he promised me that if, during the fortnight before my recital, I abstained from reciting and used my voice as little as possible and agreed to follow the treatment he prescribed, my voice by the end of that time would be normal.

I acted on his advice and accepted the engagement. After a few days I felt assured that the doctor's promise would be fulfilled, for I found that by using my voice as little as possible I gradually lost my hoarseness. When the night of my recital came, I was quite free from hoarseness, but before I was halfway through my programme, my voice was in the most distressing condition again, and by the end of the evening the hoarseness was so acute that I could hardly speak.

My disappointment was greater than I can express, for it now seemed to me that I could never look forward to more than a temporary relief, and that I should thus be forced to give up a career in which I had become deeply interested and believed I could be successful.

I saw my doctor next day and we talked the matter over, and at the end of the talk I asked him what he thought we had better do about it. 'We must go on with the treatment,' he said. I told him I could not do that, and when he asked me why, I pointed out to him that although I had faithfully carried out his instruction not to use my voice in public during his treatment, the old condition of hoarseness had returned within an hour after I started to use my voice again on the night of my recital. 'Is it not fair, then,' I asked him, 'to conclude that it was *something I was doing that evening in using my voice that was the cause of the trouble?*' He thought a moment and said 'Yes, that must be so.' 'Can you tell me, then,' I asked him, '*what it was that I did* that caused the trouble?' He frankly admitted that he could not. 'Very well,' I replied, 'if that is so, I must try and find out for myself.'

When I set out on this investigation, I had two facts to go on. I had learned by experience that reciting brought about conditions of hoarseness, and that this hoarseness tended to disappear, as long as I confined the use of my voice to ordinary speaking, and at the same time had medical treatment for my throat and vocal organs. I considered the bearing of these two facts upon my difficulty, and I saw that if ordinary speaking did not cause hoarseness while reciting did, there must be something different between what I did in reciting and what I did in ordinary speaking. If this were so, and I could find out what the difference was, it might help me to get rid of the hoarseness, and at least I could do no harm by making an experiment.

To this end I decided to make use of a mirror and observe the manner of my 'doing' both in ordinary speaking and reciting, hoping that this would enable me to distinguish the difference, if any, between them, and it seemed better to begin by watching myself during the simpler act of ordinary speaking, in order to have something to go by when I came to watch myself during the more exacting act of reciting.

Standing before a mirror I first watched myself carefully during the act of ordinary speaking. I repeated the act many times, but saw nothing in my manner of doing it that seemed wrong or unnatural. I then went on to watch myself carefully in the mirror when I recited, and I very soon noticed several things that I had not noticed when I was simply speaking. I was particularly struck by three things that I saw myself doing. I saw that as soon as I started to recite, I tended to pull back the head, depress the larynx and suck in breath through the mouth in such a way as to produce a gasping sound.

After I had noticed these tendencies I went back and watched myself again during ordinary speaking, and on this occasion I was left in little doubt that the three tendencies I had noticed for the first time when reciting were also present, though in a lesser degree, in my ordinary speaking. They were indeed so slight that I could understand why, on the previous occasions when I had watched myself in ordinary speaking,* I had altogether failed to notice them. When I discovered this

*This could hardly have been otherwise, seeing that I then lacked experience in the kind of observation necessary to enable me to detect anything wrong in the way I used myself when speaking.

marked difference between what I did in ordinary speaking and what I did in reciting, I realized that here I had a definite fact which might explain many things, and I was encouraged to go on.

I recited again and again in front of the mirror and found that the three tendencies I had already noticed became specially marked when I was reciting passages in which unusual demands were made upon my voice. This served to confirm my early suspicion that there might be some connexion between what I did with myself while reciting and my throat trouble, a not unreasonable supposition, it seemed to me, since what I did in ordinary speaking caused no noticeable harm, while what I did in reciting to meet any unusual demands on my voice brought about an acute condition of hoarseness.

From this I was led to conjecture that if pulling back my head, depressing my larynx and sucking in breath did indeed bring about a strain on my voice, it must constitute a misuse of the parts concerned. I now believed I had found the root of the trouble, for I argued that if my hoarseness arose from the way I used parts of my organism, I should get no further unless I could prevent or change this misuse.

When, however, I came to try to make practical use of this discovery, I found myself in a maze. For where was I to begin? Was it the sucking in of breath that caused the pulling back of the head and the depressing of the larynx? Or was it the pulling back of the head that caused the depressing of the larynx and the sucking in of breath? Or was it the depressing of the larynx that caused the sucking in of breath and the pulling back of the head?

As I was unable to answer these questions, all I could do was to go on patiently experimenting before the mirror. After some months I found that when reciting I could not by direct means prevent the sucking in of breath or the depressing of the larynx, but that I could to some extent prevent the pulling back of the head. This led me to a discovery which turned out to be of great importance, namely, that when I succeeded in preventing the pulling back of the head, this tended indirectly to check the sucking in of breath and the depressing of the larynx.

The importance of this discovery cannot be overestimated, for through it I was led on to the further discovery of the primary control of the working of all the mechanisms of the human organism, and this marked the first important stage of my investigation.

A further result which I also noted was that with the prevention of the misuse of these parts I tended to become less hoarse while reciting, and that as I gradually gained experience in this prevention, my liability to hoarseness tended to decrease. What is more, when, after these experiences, my throat was again examined by my medical friends, a considerable improvement was found in the general condition of my larynx and vocal cords.

In this way it was borne in upon me that the changes in *use* that I had been able to bring about by preventing the three harmful tendencies I had detected in myself had produced a marked effect upon the *functioning* of my vocal and respiratory mechanisms.

This conclusion, I now see, marked the second important stage in my investigations, for my practical experience in this specific instance brought me to realize for the first time the close connexion that exists between use and functioning.

My experience up till now had shewn me
  (1) that the tendency to put my head back was associated with my throat trouble, and
  (2) that I could relieve this trouble to a certain extent merely by preventing myself from putting my head back, since this act of prevention tended to prevent indirectly the depressing of the larynx and the sucking in of breath.
From this I argued that if I put my head definitely forward, I might be able to influence the functioning of my vocal and

respiratory mechanisms still further in the right direction, and so eradicate the tendency to hoarseness altogether. I therefore decided as my next step to put my head definitely forward, further forward, in fact, than I felt was the right thing to do.

When I came to try it, however, I found that after I had put my head forward beyond a certain point, I tended to pull it down as well as forward, and, as far as I could see, the effect of this upon my vocal and respiratory organs was much the same as when I pulled my head back and down. For in both acts there was the same depressing of the larynx that was associated with my throat trouble, and by this time I was convinced that this depressing of the larynx must be checked if my voice was ever to become normal. I therefore went on experimenting in the hope of finding some use of the head and neck which was not associated with a depressing of the larynx.

It is impossible to describe here in detail my various experiences during this long period. Suffice it to say that in the course of these experiments I came to notice that any use of my head and neck which was associated with a depressing of the larynx was also associated with a tendency to lift the chest and shorten* the stature.

As I look back I realize that this again was a discovery of far-reaching implications, and events proved that it marked a turning-point in my investigations.

This new piece of evidence suggested that the functioning of the organs of speech was influenced by my manner of using the whole torso, and that the pulling of the head back and down was not, as I had presumed, merely a misuse of the specific parts concerned, but one that was inseparably bound up with a misuse of other mechanisms which involved the act of shortening the stature. If this were so, it would clearly be useless to expect such improvement as I needed from merely

*Although it would probably be more correct to use the phrases '*increase* the stature', '*decrease* the stature', I have decided to use the phrases 'lengthen the stature', 'shorten the stature', because the words 'lengthen' and 'shorten' are those most commonly used in this connexion.

preventing the wrong use of the head and neck. I realized that I must also prevent those other associated wrong uses which brought about the shortening of the stature.

This led me on to a long series of experiments in some of which I attempted to prevent the shortening of the stature, in others actually to lengthen it, noting the results in each case. For a time I alternated between these two forms of experiment, and after noting the effect of each upon my voice, I found that the best conditions of my larynx and vocal mechanisms and the least tendency to hoarseness were associated with a *lengthening* of the stature. Unfortunately, I found that when I came to practise, I shortened far more than I lengthened, and when I came to look for an explanation of this, I saw that it was due to my tendency to pull my head down as I tried to put it forward in order to lengthen. After further experimentation I found at last that in order to maintain a lengthening of the stature it was necessary that my head should tend to go upwards, not downwards, when I put it forward; in short, that to lengthen I *must put my head forward and up*.

As is shewn by what follows, this proved to be the primary control of my use in all my activities.

When, however, I came to try to put my head forward and up *while reciting*, I noticed that my old tendency to lift the chest increased, and that with this went a tendency to increase the arch of the spine and thus bring about what I now call a 'narrowing of the back'. This, I saw, had an adverse effect on the shape and functioning of the torso itself, and I therefore concluded that to maintain a lengthening it was not sufficient to put my head forward and up, but that I must put it forward and up in such a way that I prevented the lifting of the chest and simultaneously brought about a widening of the back.

Having got so far, I considered I should now be justified in attempting to put these findings into practice. To this end I proceeded in my vocal work to try to prevent my old habit of pulling my head back and down and lifting the chest (shortening the stature), and to combine this act of prevention with an attempt to put the head forward and up (lengthening the stature) and widen the back. This was my first attempt to combine 'prevention' and 'doing' in one activity, and I never for a moment doubted that I should be able to do this, but I found that although I was now able to put the head forward and up and widen the back as acts in themselves, *I could not maintain these conditions in speaking or reciting.*

This made me suspicious that I was not doing what I thought I was doing, and I decided once more to bring the mirror to my aid. Later on I took into use two additional mirrors, one on each side of the central one, and with their aid I found that my suspicions were justified. For there I saw that at the critical moment when I tried to combine the prevention of shortening with a positive attempt to *maintain a lengthening and speak at the same time,* I did not put my head forward and up as I intended, but actually put it back. Here then was startling proof that I was doing the opposite of what I believed I was doing and of what I had decided I ought to do.

I break my story here to draw attention to a very curious fact, even though it tells against myself. My reader will remember that in my earlier experiments, when I wished to make certain of what I was doing with myself in the familiar act of reciting, I had derived invaluable help from the use of a mirror. Despite this past experience and the knowledge that I had gained from it, I now set out on an experiment which brought into play a new use of certain parts and involved sensory experiences that were totally unfamiliar, without its even occurring to me that for this purpose I should need the help of the mirror more than ever.

This shews how confident I was, in spite of my past experience, that I should be able to put into practice any idea that I thought desirable. When I found myself unable to do so, I thought that this was merely a personal idiosyncrasy, but my teaching experience of the past thirty-five years and my observation of people with whom I have come into contact in other ways have convinced me that this was not an idiosyn-

crasy, but that most people would have done the same in similar circumstances. I was indeed suffering from a delusion that is practically universal, the delusion that because we are able to do what we 'will to do' in acts that are habitual and involve familiar sensory experiences, we shall be equally successful in doing what we 'will to do' in acts which are contrary to our habit and therefore involve sensory experiences that are unfamiliar.

When I realized this, I was much disturbed and I saw that the whole situation would have to be reconsidered. I went back to the beginning again, to my original conclusion that the cause of my throat trouble was to be found in something I was doing myself when I used my voice. I had since discovered both what this 'something' was and what I believed I ought to do instead, if my vocal organs were to function properly. But this had not helped me much, for when the time came for me to apply what I had learned to my reciting, and I had tried to do what I ought to do, I had failed. Obviously, then, my next step was to find out at what point in my 'doing' I had gone wrong.

There was nothing for it but to persevere, and I practised patiently month after month, as I had been doing hitherto, with varying experiences of success and failure, but without much enlightenment. In time, however, I profited by these experiences, for through them I came to see that any attempt to maintain my lengthening when reciting not only involved on my part the prevention of the wrong use of certain specific parts and the substitution of what I believed to be a better use of these parts, but that this attempt also involved my bringing into play the use of all those parts of the organism required for the activities incident to the act of reciting, such as standing, walking, using the arms or hands for gesture, interpretation, etc.

Observation in the mirror shewed me that when I was standing to recite I was using these other parts in certain wrong ways which synchronized with my wrong way of using my head and neck, larynx, vocal and breathing organs, and which involved a condition of undue muscle tension throughout my organism. I observed that this condition of undue muscle tension affected particularly the use of my legs, feet and toes, my toes being contracted and bent downwards in such a way that my feet were unduly arched, my weight thrown more on to the outside of my feet than it should have been, and my balance interfered with.

On discovering this, I thought back to see if I could account for it, and I recalled an instruction that had been given to me in the past by the late Mr James Cathcart (at one time a member of Mr Charles Kean's Company) when I was taking lessons from him in dramatic expression and interpretation. Not being pleased with my way of standing and walking, he would say to me from time to time, 'Take hold of the floor with your feet.' He would then proceed to shew me what he meant by this, and I did my best to copy him, believing that if I was told what to do to correct something that was wrong, I should be able to do it and all would be well. I persevered and in time believed that my way of standing was now satisfactory, because I thought I was 'taking hold of the floor with my feet' as I had seen him do.

The belief is very generally held that if only we are told what to do in order to correct a wrong way of doing something, we can do it, and that if we feel we are doing it, all is well. All my experience, however, goes to shew that this belief is a delusion.

On recalling this experience I continued with the aid of mirrors to observe the use of myself more carefully than ever, and came to realize that what I was doing with my legs, feet and toes when standing to recite was exerting a most harmful general influence upon the use of myself throughout my organism. This convinced me that the use of these parts involved an abnormal amount of muscle tension and was indirectly associated with my throat trouble, and I was strengthened in this conviction when I reminded myself that my teacher had found it necessary in the past to try and improve my way of standing in order to get better results in my reciting. It gradually dawned upon me that the wrong way I was using myself when I thought I was 'taking hold of the floor with my feet' was the same wrong way I was using myself when in reciting I pulled my head back, depressed my larynx, etc, and that this wrong way of using myself constituted a combined wrong use of the whole of my physical–mental mechanisms. I then realized that this was the use which I habitually brought into play for all my activities, that it was what I may call the 'habitual use' of myself, and that my desire to recite, like any other stimulus to activity, would inevitably cause this habitual wrong use to come into play and dominate any attempt I might be making to employ a better use of myself in reciting.

The influence of this wrong use was bound to be strong because of its being habitual, but in my case it was greatly strengthened because during the past years I had undoubtedly been cultivating it through my efforts to carry out my teacher's instructions to 'take hold of the floor with my feet' when I recited. The influence of this *cultivated* habitual use, therefore, acted as an almost irresistible stimulus to me to use myself in the wrong way I was accustomed to; this stimulus to general wrong use was far stronger than the stimulus of my desire to employ the new use of my head and neck, and I now saw that it was this influence which led me, as soon as I stood up to recite, to put my head in the opposite direction to that which I desired. I now had proof of one thing at least, that all my efforts up till now to improve the use of myself in reciting had been misdirected.

It is important to remember that the use of a specific part in any activity is closely associated with the use of other parts of the organism, and that the influence exerted by the various parts one upon another is continuously changing in accordance with the manner of use of these parts. If a part directly employed in the activity is being used in a comparatively new way which is still unfamiliar, the stimulus to use this part in the new way is weak in comparison with the stimulus to use the

*other parts of the organism, which are being indirectly
employed in the activity, in the old habitual way.*

*In the present case, an attempt was being made to bring
about an unfamiliar use of the head and neck for the purpose
of reciting. The stimulus to employ the new use of the head and
neck was therefore bound to be weak as compared with the
stimulus to employ the wrong habitual use of the feet and legs
which had become familiar through being cultivated in the act
of reciting.*

*Herein lies the difficulty in making changes from un-
satisfactory to satisfactory conditions of use and functioning,
and my teaching experience has taught me that when a wrong
habitual use has been cultivated in a person for whatever
purpose, its influence in the early stages of the lessons is
practically irresistible.*

This led me to a long consideration of the whole question of
the direction* of the use of myself. 'What is this direction,' I
asked myself, 'upon which I have been depending?' I had to
admit that I had never thought out how I directed the use of
myself, but that I used myself habitually in the way that *felt
natural* to me. In other words, I like everyone else depended
upon 'feeling' for the direction of my use. Judging, however,
from the results of my experiments, this method of direction
had led me into error (as, for instance, when I put my head
back when I intended to put it forward and up), proving that
the 'feeling' associated with this direction of my use was
untrustworthy.

This indeed was a blow. If ever anyone was in an impasse, it
was I. For here I was, faced with the fact that my feeling, the
only guide I had to depend upon for the direction of my use,
was untrustworthy. At the time I believed that this was

*When I employ the words 'direction' and 'directed' with 'use' in such
phrases as 'direction of my use' and 'I directed the use', etc, I wish to
indicate the process involved in projecting messages from the brain to the
mechanisms and in conducting the energy necessary to the use of these
mechanisms.

peculiar to myself, and that my case was exceptional because of the continuous ill-health I had experienced for as long as I could remember, but as soon as I tested other people to see whether they were using themselves in the way they thought they were, I found that the feeling by which they directed the use of themselves was also untrustworthy, indeed, that the only difference in this regard between them and myself was one of degree. Discouraged as I was, however, I refused to believe that the problem was hopeless. I began to see that my findings up till now implied the possibility of the opening up of an entirely new field of enquiry, and I was obsessed with the desire to explore it. 'Surely,' I argued, 'if it is possible for feeling to become untrustworthy as a means of direction, it should also be possible to make it trustworthy again.'

The idea of the wonderful potentialities of man had been a source of inspiration to me ever since I had come to know Shakespeare's great word picture:

> What a piece of work is a man! how noble in reason! how infinite in faculty! in form and moving how express and admirable! in action how like an angel! in apprehension how like a god! the beauty of the world! the paragon of animals!

But these words seemed to me now to be contradicted by what I had discovered in myself and others. For what could be less 'noble in reason', less 'infinite in faculty' than that man, despite his potentialities, should have fallen into such error in the use of himself, and in this way brought about such a lowering in his standard of functioning that in everything he attempts to accomplish, these harmful conditions tend to become more and more exaggerated? In consequence, how many people are there today of whom it may be said, as regards their use of themselves, 'in form and moving how express and admirable'? Can we any longer consider man in this regard 'the paragon of animals'?

I can remember at this period discussing with my father the errors in use which I had noticed both in myself and in others, and contending that in this respect there was no difference between us and the dog or cat. When he asked me why, I replied, 'Because we do not *know* how we use ourselves any more than the dog or cat *knows*'. By this I meant that man's direction of his use, through being based upon feeling, was as unreasoned and instinctive as that of the animal.* I refer to this conversation as shewing that I had already realized that in our present state of civilization which calls for continuous and rapid adaptation to a quickly changing environment, the unreasoned, instinctive direction of use such as meets the needs of the cat or dog was no longer sufficient to meet human

*It may be contended that the athlete who successfully performs a complicated feat does consciously control his movements. It is true, of course, that in a great many cases he is able by practice on the 'trial and error' plan to acquire an automatic proficiency in performing the specific movements necessary for this feat, but this does not in any way prove that he is controlling these movements consciously. And even in those rare instances where the athlete consciously controls and co-ordinates certain specific movements, it still cannot be said that he consciously controls the use of himself as a whole in his performance. For it is safe to conclude that he does not *know* what use of his mechanisms as a whole is the best possible for making the specific movements he desires, so that should anything happen, as it often does, to cause a change in the familiar habitual use of his mechanisms, his proficiency in making these specific movements will also be interfered with. Practical experience shews that once he has lost this original standard of proficiency, he cannot easily regain it, and this is not surprising seeing that he lacks the knowledge of how to direct the general use of himself which alone would enable him to restore the familiar use of his mechanisms which gave him his proficiency. (In this connexion, many cases have been known of people who, having purposely imitated the peculiarities of a stutterer, have themselves developed the habit of stuttering, and in spite of all their efforts have failed to regain their original standard of proficiency in speaking.)

Because he lacks this knowledge, the athlete, like the animal, has to depend upon his feeling for the direction of the working of his mechanisms, and as that feeling has become more or less untrustworthy in the majority of athletes (a fact that can be demonstrated), the mechanisms which he employs for his activities are bound to be misdirected. Such direction, being as unreasoned as that of the animal, cannot be compared with that conscious reasoned direction which is associated with a primary control of the mechanisms of the self as a working unity.

needs. I had proved in my own case and in that of others that instinctive control and direction of use had become so unsatisfactory, and the associated feeling so untrustworthy as a guide, that it could lead us to do the very opposite of what we wished to do or thought we were doing. If, then, as I suspected, this untrustworthiness of feeling was a product of civilized life, it would tend, as time went on, to become more and more a universal menace, in which case a knowledge of the means whereby trustworthiness could be restored to feeling would be invaluable. I saw that the search for this knowledge would open out an entirely new field of exploration and one that promised more than any that I had yet heard of, and I began to reconsider my own difficulties in the light of this new fact.

Certain points impressed themselves particularly upon me:

(1) that the pulling of my head back and down, when I *felt* that I was putting it forward and up, was proof that the use of the specific parts concerned was being misdirected, and that this misdirection was associated with untrustworthy feeling;

(2) that this misdirection was instinctive, and, together with the associated untrustworthy feeling, was part and parcel of my habitual use of myself;

(3) that this instinctive misdirection leading to wrong habitual use of myself, including most noticeably the wrong use of my head and neck, *came into play as the result of a decision to use my voice; this misdirection, in other words, was my instinctive response (reaction) to the stimulus to use my voice.*

When I came to consider the significance of this last point, it occurred to me that if, when the stimulus came to me to use my voice, I could inhibit the misdirection associated with the wrong habitual use of my head and neck, I should be stopping off at its source my unsatisfactory reaction to the idea of reciting, which expressed itself in pulling back the head, depressing the larynx, and sucking in breath. Once this misdirection was inhibited, my next step would be to discover what direction would be necessary to ensure a new and improved use of the head and neck, and, indirectly, of the larynx and breathing and other mechanisms, for I believed that such direction, when put into practice, would ensure a satisfactory instead of an unsatisfactory reaction to the stimulus to use my voice.

In the work that followed I came to see that to get a direction of my use which would *ensure* this satisfactory reaction, I must cease to rely upon the feeling associated with my instinctive direction, and in its place employ my reasoning processes, in order

(1) to analyse the conditions of use present;

(2) to select (reason out) the means whereby a more satisfactory use could be brought about;

(3) to project *consciously* the directions required for putting these means into effect.

In short, I concluded that if I were ever to be able to react satisfactorily to the stimulus to use my voice, I must replace my old instinctive (unreasoned) direction of myself by a new conscious (reasoned) direction.

The idea of taking the control of the use of the mechanisms of the human creature from the instinctive on to the conscious plane has already been justified by the results which have been obtained by applying it in practice, but it may be many years before its true significance as a factor in human development is fully recognized.

I set out to put this idea into practice, but I was at once brought up short by a series of startling and unexpected experiences. Like most people, I had believed up to this moment that if I thought out carefully how to improve my way of performing a certain act, I should be guided by my reasoning rather than by my feeling when it came to putting this thought into action, and that my 'mind' was the superior and more effective directing agent. But the fallacy of this became apparent to me as soon as I attempted to employ conscious direction for the purpose of correcting some wrong use of myself which was habitual and therefore *felt right* to me. In actual practice I found that there was no clear dividing line between my unreasoned and my reasoned direction of myself, and that I was quite unable to prevent the two from overlapping. I was successful in employing my reasoning up to the point of projecting the directions which, after analysing the conditions of use present, I had decided were required for the new and improved use, and all went well as long as I did not attempt to carry these directions out for the purpose of speaking. For instance, as soon as any stimulus reached me to use my voice, and I tried in response to *do* the new thing which my conscious direction should bring about (such as putting the head forward and up), and *speak at the same time*, I found I immediately reverted to all my old wrong habits of use (such as putting my head back, etc). There was no question about this. I could see it actually happening in the mirror. This was clear proof that at the critical moment when I attempted to gain my end by means which were contrary to those associated with my old habits of use, my instinctive direction dominated my reasoning direction. It dominated my will to do what I had decided was the right thing to do, and although I was trying (as we understand 'trying') to do it. Over and over again I had the experience that immediately the stimulus to speak came to me, I invariably responded by doing something according to my old habitual use associated with the act of speaking.

After many disappointing experiences of this kind I decided to give up any attempt for the present to 'do' anything to gain my end, and I came to see at last that if I was ever to be able to change my habitual use and dominate my instinctive direction, *it would be necessary for me to make the experience of receiving the stimulus to speak and of refusing to do anything immediately in response*. For I saw that an immediate response was the result of a decision on my part to do something *at once*, to go directly for a certain end, and by acting quickly on this decision I did not give myself the opportunity to project as many times as was necessary the new directions which I had reasoned out were the best means whereby I could attain that end. This meant that the old instinctive direction which, associated with untrustworthy feeling, had been the controlling factor up to that moment in the building up of my wrong habitual use, still controlled the *manner* of my response, with the inevitable result that my old wrong habitual use was again and again brought into play.

I therefore decided to confine my work to giving myself the directions for the new 'means-whereby',* instead of actually trying to 'do' them or to relate them to the 'end' of speaking. I would give the new directions in front of the mirror for long periods together, for successive days and weeks and sometimes even months, without attempting to 'do' them, and the experience I gained in giving these directions proved of great value when the time came for me to consider how to put them into practice.

This experience taught me

(1) that before attempting to 'do' even the first part of the new 'means-whereby' which I had decided to employ in order to gain my end (ie, vocal use and reciting), I must give the directions preparatory to the doing of this first part very many times;

(2) that I must *continue* to give the directions preparatory to the doing of the first part while I gave the directions preparatory to the doing of the second part;

(3) that I must *continue* to give the directions preparatory to the doing of the first and second parts while I gave the directions preparatory to the doing of the third part; and so on for the doing of the fourth and other parts as required.

Lastly, I discovered that after I had become familiar with the combined process of giving the directions for the new

*The phrase 'means-whereby' will be used throughout this book to indicate the reasoned means to the gaining of an end. These means included the inhibition of the habitual use of the mechanisms of the organism, and the conscious projection of new directions necessary to the performance of the different acts involved in a new and more satisfactory use of these mechanisms.

'means-whereby' in their sequence and of employing the various corresponding mechanisms in order to bring about the new use, I must continue this process in my practice for a considerable time before actually attempting to employ the new 'means-whereby' for the purpose of speaking.

The process I have just described is an example of what Professor John Dewey has called 'thinking in activity', and anyone who carries it out faithfully while trying to gain an end will find that he is acquiring a new experience in what he calls 'thinking'. My daily teaching experience shews me that in working for a given end, we can all project one direction, but to continue to give this direction as we project the second, and to continue to give these two while we add a third, and to continue to keep the three directions going as we proceed to gain the end, has proved to be the pons asinorum of every pupil I have so far known.*

The time came when I believed I had practised the 'means-whereby' long enough, and I started to try and employ them for the purpose of speaking, but to my dismay I found that I failed far more often than I succeeded. The further I went with these attempts, the more perplexing the situation became, for I was certainly attempting to inhibit my habitual response to the stimulus to speak, and I had certainly given the new directions over and over again. At least, this is what I had intended to do and thought I had done, so that, as far as I could then see, I should have been able to employ the new 'means-whereby' for the gaining of my end with some degree of confidence. The fact remained that I failed more often than not, and nothing was more certain than that I must go back and reconsider my premises.

This reconsideration shewed me more clearly than ever that the occasions when I failed were those on which I was unable to prevent the dominance of my wrong habitual use, as I

---

*The phrase 'all together, one after the other' expresses the idea of combined activity I wish to convey here.

attempted to employ the new 'means-whereby' with the idea of gaining my end and speaking. I also saw (and this was of the utmost importance) that, in spite of all my preliminary work, the instinctive direction associated with my habitual use still dominated my conscious reasoning direction. So confident was I, however, that the new means I had chosen were right for my purpose, that I decided I must look elsewhere for the cause of my unsatisfactory results. In time I began to doubt whether perhaps my failures were not due to some shortcoming in myself, and that I personally was unable to do a thing with satisfactory 'means-whereby' when someone else might have been successful. I looked all round for any other possible causes of failure, and after a long period of investigation I came to the conclusion that it was necessary for me to seek some concrete proof whether, at the critical moment when I attempted to gain my end and speak, I was really continuing to project the directions in their proper sequence for the employment of the new and more satisfactory use, as I thought I was, or whether I was reverting to the instinctive misdirection of my old habitual use which had been associated with all my throat trouble. By careful experimentation I discovered that I gave my directions for the new use in their sequence right up to the point when I tried to gain my end and speak, but that, at the critical moment when persistence in giving the new directions would have brought success, I reverted instead to the misdirection associated with my old wrong habitual use. This was concrete proof that I was not continuing to project my directions for the new use for the purpose of speaking, as I thought I was, but that my reaction to the stimulus to speak was still my instinctive reaction through my habitual use. Clearly, to 'feel' or think I had inhibited the old instinctive reaction was no proof that I had really done so, and I must find some way of 'knowing'.

I had already noticed that on the occasions when I failed, the instinctive misdirection associated with my old habitual use always dominated my reasoning direction for the new use, and I gradually car   to see that this could hardly be otherwise.

Ever since the beginning of man's growth and development
the only form of direction of the use of himself of which he
has had any experience has been instinctive direction, which
might in this sense be called a racial inheritance. Was it then
to be wondered at that in my case the influence of this
inherited instinctive direction associated with my old habitual use had rendered futile most of my efforts to employ a
conscious, reasoning direction for a new use, especially when
the use of myself which was associated with instinctive
direction had become so familiar that it was now part and
parcel of me, and so *felt right and natural*? In trying to
employ a conscious, reasoning direction to bring about a new
use, I was therefore combating in myself not only that racial
tendency which causes us all at critical moments to revert to
instinctive direction and so to the familiar use of ourselves
that feels right, but also a racial inexperience in projecting
conscious directions at all, and particularly conscious directions in sequence.

As the reader knows, I had recognized much earlier that I
ought not to trust to my feeling for the direction of my use,
but I had never fully realized all that this implied, namely,
that the sensory experience associated with the new use
would be so unfamiliar and therefore 'feel' so unnatural and
wrong that I, like everyone else, with my ingrained habit of
judging whether experiences of use were 'right' or not by the
way they *felt*, would almost inevitably balk at employing the
new use. Obviously, any new use must feel different from
the old, and if the old use felt right, the new use was bound to
feel wrong. I now had to face the fact that in all my attempts
during these past months I had been trying to employ a new
use of myself which was bound to feel wrong, at the same
time trusting to my feeling of what was right to tell me
whether I was employing it or not. This meant that all my
efforts up till now had resolved themselves into an attempt to
employ a reasoning direction of my use at the moment of
speaking, while for the purpose of this attempt I was actually
bringing into play my old habitual use and so reverting to my

instinctive misdirection. Small wonder that this attempt had proved futile!

Faced with this, I now saw that if I was ever to succeed in making the changes in use I desired, I must subject the processes directing my use to a new experience, the experience, that is, of being dominated by reasoning instead of by feeling, particularly at the critical moment when the giving of directions merged into 'doing' for the gaining of the end I had decided upon. This meant that I must be prepared to carry on with any procedure I had reasoned out as best for my purpose, even though that procedure might *feel wrong*. In other words, my trust in my reasoning processes to bring me safely to my 'end' must be a genuine trust, not a half-trust needing the assurance of *feeling right* as well. I must at all costs work out some plan by which to obtain concrete proof that my instinctive reaction to the stimulus to gain my end *remained inhibited*, while I projected in their sequence the directions for the employment of the new use at the critical moment of gaining that end.

After making many attempts to solve this problem and gaining experience which proved to be of great value and interest to me, I finally adopted the following plan.*

Supposing that the 'end' I decided to work for was to speak a certain sentence, I would start in the same way as before and

(1) inhibit any immediate response to the stimulus to speak the sentence,

(2) project in their sequence the directions for the primary control which I had reasoned out as being best for the purpose of bringing about the new and improved use of myself in speaking, and

(3) continue to project these directions until I believed I was sufficiently *au fait* with them to employ them for the purpose of gaining my end and speaking the sentence.

At this moment, the moment that had always proved critical for me because it was then that I tended to revert to my wrong

*This plan, though simple in theory, has proved difficult for most pupils to put into practice.

habitual use, I would change my usual procedure and

(4) *while still continuing to project the directions for the new use* I would stop and consciously reconsider my first decision, and ask myself 'Shall I after all go on to gain the end I have decided upon and speak the sentence? Or shall I not? Or shall I go on to gain some other end altogether?' — *and then and there make a fresh decision,*

(5) either

not to gain my original end, in which case *I would continue to project the directions for maintaining the new use* and not go on to speak the sentence;

or

to change my end and do something different, say, lift my hand instead of speaking the sentence, in which case *I would continue to project the directions for maintaining the new use* to carry out this last decision and lift my hand;

or

to go on after all and gain my original end, in which case *I would continue to project the directions for maintaining the new use* to speak the sentence.

It will be seen that under this new plan the change in procedure came at the critical moment when hitherto, in going on to gain my end, I had so often reverted to instinctive misdirection and my wrong habitual use. I reasoned that if I stopped at that moment and then, *without ceasing to project the directions for the new use,* decided afresh to what end the new use should be employed, I should by this procedure be subjecting my instinctive processes of direction to an experience contrary to any experience in which they had hitherto been drilled. Up to that time the stimulus of a decision to gain a certain end had always resulted in the same habitual activity, involving the projection of the instinctive directions for the use which I habitually employed for the gaining of that end. By this new procedure, *as long as the reasoned directions for the bringing about of new conditions of use were consciously maintained,* the stimulus of a decision to gain a certain end would result in an activity differing from the old habitual activity, in that the old activity could not be controlled outside the gaining of a given end, whereas the new activity could be controlled for the gaining of any end that was consciously desired.

I would point out that this procedure is contrary, not only to any procedure in which our individual instinctive direction has been drilled, but contrary also to that in which man's instinctive processes have been drilled continuously all through his evolutionary experience.

When I came to work on this plan, I found that this reasoning was borne out by experience. For by actually deciding, in the majority of cases, to maintain my new conditions of use either to gain some end other than the one originally decided upon, or simply to refuse to gain the original end, I obtained at last the concrete proof I was looking for, namely, that my instinctive response to the stimulus to gain my original end was not only inhibited at the start, *but remained inhibited right through, whilst my directions for the new use were being projected.* And the experience I gained in maintaining the new manner of use while going on to gain some other end or refusing to gain my original end, helped me to maintain the new use on those occasions when I decided at the critical moment to go on after all and gain my original end and speak the sentence. This was further proof that I was becoming able to defeat any influence of that habitual wrong use in speaking to which my original decision to 'speak the sentence' had been the stimulus, and that my conscious, reasoning direction was at last dominating the unreasoning, instinctive direction associated with my unsatisfactory habitual use of myself.

After I had worked on this plan for a considerable time, I became free from my tendency to revert to my wrong habitual use in reciting, and the marked effect of this upon my functioning convinced me that I was at last on the right track, for once free from this tendency, I also became free from the throat and vocal trouble and from the respiratory and nasal difficulties with which I had been beset from birth.

CHAPTER II

Use and Functioning in Relation to Reaction

The reader who reviews the experiences that I have tried to set down in the previous chapter will notice that at a certain point in my investigation I came to realize that my reaction to a particular stimulus was constantly the opposite of that which I desired, and that in my search for the cause of this, I discovered that my sensory appreciation (feeling) of the use of my mechanisms was so untrustworthy that it led me to react by means of a use of myself which *felt* right, but was, in fact, too often wrong for my purpose.

I draw attention to this point, because over the long period of years in which I have been engaged in teaching pupils to improve and control the manner of their use of themselves, I have found that untrustworthiness of sensory appreciation is present in varying degrees in all of them, exerting, as in my own case, a harmful influence upon their use and functioning, and consequently upon their manner of reacting to stimuli. The whole experience, indeed, convinces me that the prevalence of sensory untrustworthiness is of the utmost significance in relation to the problem of the control of human reaction.

Another point of importance in relation to the control of human reaction is that it was through my discovery of the primary control that I was able to bring about the improvement in the sensory appreciation of the use of my mechanisms which was associated with the improvement in functioning throughout my organism. By the time I had reached the stage when a new manner of use had become established through my conscious employment of this primary control, I was able, when the stimulus came to me to use my voice to recite, to inhibit my instinctive misdirection leading to the old harmful use of my head and neck and vocal organs, and so to my hoarseness, and to substitute for it a conscious direction leading to a new use of my head, neck and vocal organs which was not associated with hoarseness.

This meant that the stimulus to use my voice no longer brought into play the old reflex activity which included the pulling of my head back and down, leading to a shortening of my stature, and which constituted my harmful habitual reaction to that stimulus, but instead, a new reflex activity which included putting my head forward and up to lengthen the stature and which, by its results, proved to be a satisfactory reaction to that stimulus.

That fact that I was able, through my employment of the primary control, to bring about such an improvement in my reaction to the stimulus to use my voice that vocal activity did not result in hoarseness, is proof that quite early in my experiences a practical means had been found, whereby my habitual reflex activity was 'conditioned' as a natural consequence of the procedure adopted, since the new reflex activity to which it was changed *in the process* was associated with new and improved general conditions of use and functioning.*

Indeed, the results that have been obtained by adopting the procedure described on pages 45-48 furnish evidence of how harmful reflex activity brought about by misdirection of use can be consciously held in check, even in face of the excitation

*In this connexion the following quotation from a paper read by Dr A. Murdoch, of Bexhill-on-Sea, at the St Andrews (James Mackenzie) Institute on March 6, 1928, may be of interest: 'Mr Alexander has built up the theory on which he has based his practice from the observation of the movements of the body as a whole, and he has made use of lost or unused associated involuntary reflexes with a rare insight, and by recreating them into new conditioned reflexes he has laid the foundation for a new outlook on disease and its diagnosis and treatment.'

involved in carrying out the procedure.*

More than this, my experience has shewn that in cases where the knowledge of how to direct the primary control has led to a change for the better in the manner of the use of the mechanisms throughout the organism, the results of this 'conditioning' can safely be left to take their own form. As Professor John Dewey writes, 'Science is, after all, a matter of perfected skill in conducting enquiry ... not "something finished, absolute in itself," but the result of a certain technique.'†

Seeing, therefore, that it proved possible to bring about a conscious control of my reaction through a change in the direction of my use, the reader will understand why, in my opinion, *the substitution of conscious for instinctive direction in the changing of use* is of primary importance, and why I believe a knowledge of the means whereby this change can be brought about would be of inestimable value in all educational work.

The experiences I gained in dealing with my own difficulties have proved of the greatest value to me in dealing practically with the difficulties and requirements of my pupils. First and foremost, I learned from these experiences that I could not enable my pupils to control the functioning of their organs, systems or reflexes *directly*, but that by teaching them to employ consciously the primary control of their use I could put them in command of the means whereby their functioning generally can be *indirectly* controlled. My adoption of this principle in the employment of my technique has been fully justified by experience, and I have had no reason up till now for departing from it. Indeed, my continued experience convinces me that unless the building up of a conscious direction of use, in association with an improving standard of sensory apprec-

---

*According to this procedure the subject starts by consciously projecting the directions for the means whereby he will gain a certain end, and, at the critical moment of going on to gain this end, makes a fresh decision as to whether he will employ these 'means-whereby' to gain the original end or some other.

†*Experience and Nature* (Open Court Publishing Co., 1926).

iation of that use, is made the primary consideration of all those who, in different spheres, are dealing with the problem of the control of human reaction, we are not likely to develop a method for meeting the problem of the control of conscious, or, as it is sometimes called, 'conditioned' behaviour.

In any discussion of human reaction certain well-known facts about the nature of human activity may be taken as premises.

Human activity is primarily a process of reacting unceasingly to stimuli received from within or without the self. The first breath taken by a newly born child is a reaction to a stimulus to the respiratory centre, and the child remains a living organism only so long as it is capable of receiving stimuli and of reacting to them. No human being can receive a stimulus except through the sensory mechanisms, and supposing one could prevent the sensory mechanisms from receiving a stimulus, no reaction would be possible and therefore no further activity. Life itself would then cease.

When once it is recognized that every act is a reaction to a stimulus received through the sensory mechanisms, no act can be described as wholly 'mental' or wholly 'physical'. The most that can be said is that in some acts the 'mental' side predominates and in others the 'physical'. For instance, let us take the act of lifting the arm, which would be described offhand by many people as a 'physical' act. If we consider what happens between the receipt of a stimulus to lift the arm and the performance of the act, we shall see that a concerted activity takes place which brings into play not only the processes which most people are accustomed to regard as 'physical', but also the processes which they regard as 'mental'. The result of the receipt of a stimulus to lift the arm is, as we all know, a 'mental' conception of the act of lifting the arm, this conception being followed by another so-called 'mental' process, that of giving or withholding consent to react to the stimulus to lift the arm. If this consent is withheld, the reaction which would result in a lifting of the arm is inhibited, and the arm is not lifted. If consent is given, the direction of the mechanisms required for the act of lifting the arm becomes operative, and messages are sent out which bring about the contraction of certain groups of muscles and the relaxation of others, and the arm is lifted.

But in this connexion it is of the utmost importance to remember that in most people their direction of the use of themselves is habitual and instinctive, so that once consent has been given to react to the stimulus to perform a certain act, they will perform that act, as we say, 'instinctively', that is, without any reasoned conception of what direction of the use of the mechanisms is required for its satisfactory performance.

Unfortunately, with the increasing prevalence of untrustworthy sensory appreciation,* this instinctive direction of use tends, as time goes on, to become more and more a misdirection, having a harmful effect, as was proved in my own case, upon functioning and, consequently, upon the reactions which result.

These unsatisfactory reactions manifest themselves as symptoms of defect, of so-called 'mental' or 'moral' failing, disorder and disease, and their presence may therefore be taken as an indication of the presence also of wrong use and functioning† throughout the organism. My experience with cases manifesting any such 'symptoms' has shewn me that where a new and satisfactory direction of the use of the mechanisms has been brought about, leading to an improvement in the associated functioning, these symptoms tend gradually to disappear in the process, and to be replaced by symptoms of health and wellbeing, or satisfactory reactions. For this reason I claim that the primary requirement in dealing with all specific symptoms is to prevent the misdirection which leads to wrong use and

---

*This is a fact which came to light in my investigations (see Chapter I, pp. 35 and 36) and is one that can be demonstrated.

†I wish to make it plain that whenever I use the phrase 'use and functioning' in relation to the human organism, I do not indicate by it mechanical activity as such, but include in the phrase all manifestations of human activity involved in what we designate as conception or understanding, withholding or giving consent, thinking, reasoning, directing, etc. For the manifestation of such activities cannot be dissociated from the use of the mechanisms and the associated functioning of the organism.

functioning, and to establish in its place a new and satisfactory direction as a means of bringing about an improvement in use and functioning throughout the organism.

This indirect procedure is true to the principle that the unity of the human organism is indivisible, and where there is an understanding of the means whereby the use of the mechanisms can be directed in practice as a concerted activity, in the sense I have tried to define, the principle of unity works for good. But there is a reverse side to the picture. It is in the nature of unity that any change in a part means a change in the whole, and the parts of the human organism are knit so closely into a unity that any attempt to make a fundamental change in the working of a part is bound to alter the use and adjustment of the whole. This means that where the concerted use of the mechanisms of the organism is faulty, any attempt to eradicate a defect otherwise than by changing and improving this faulty concerted use is bound to throw out the balance somewhere else.*

This danger is seldom recognized by those who have to diagnose and deal with cases of ailment or disability, but I am prepared to demonstrate that *in the process* of 'curing' a wrong symptom by specific treatment, even though this treatment may be outwardly successful, other less easily recognized but often more harmful defects are brought about in other parts of the organism. It is the old story of the seven devils.†

---

*See Chapter IV, pp. 77 and 78.

†In this connexion it is very interesting to compare what Sir E. Holderness, the well-known authority on golf, wrote in the *Evening Standard* of March 17, 1928.

'Here is a true tale of a friend. He suffered from a chronic slice, and in despair went to a professional who offered him an easy cure by making him put his left hand on the top of the club and his right hand underneath. Then he told him to bang away with confidence. Wonderful to relate, the slice disappeared and for one afternoon he drove divinely. But where there had been one devil, seven worse ones came in its place; and for weeks and months he endured the agony of pulls and smothers. His last state was more pitiful than his first.'

The results of my teaching work have shewn me that no diagnosis can be complete which is not based on that principle of the unity in working of the mechanisms of the organism which involves a close connexion between the manner of use of the mechanisms and the standard of functioning throughout the organism.

In what follows I shall bring forward several illustrations to shew how experts in widely differing spheres of activity fail to recognize this principle in their practical dealings with those who consult them with a view to correcting some defect or disability, and how this leads to an incomplete diagnosis and seriously limits the scope of the adviser, whatever his line.

A fair judgment of any procedure can only be reached by an examination of the principle on which it is founded. Where the principle is unsound, the procedure must fail in the long run. I therefore wish the practical procedures which I am now putting forward to be judged by the principle which underlies them.

CHAPTER III

The Golfer Who Cannot Keep his
Eyes on the Ball

Let us suppose that a golfer who does not make a success of his golf consults a professional with a view to improving his play. After watching him play, the professional tells him among other things that he is taking his eyes off the ball, and impresses on him that if he wishes to improve his stroke, he *must* keep his eyes on the ball. The golfer starts to play with every intention of following out his teacher's instructions, but finds that in spite of all his efforts, he still takes his eyes off the ball.

There are several points in this situation that could be discussed, but I wish, in this chapter, to confine my consideration to the principle which underlies not only the teacher's diagnosis and instructions, but also the procedure of the pupil when he decides to carry the instructions out.

Certain questions at once suggest themselves.

Why does the golfer take his eyes off the ball in the first place, when according to the experts he should not do so?

Why does he *continue* to take his eyes off the ball after he has decided to keep them *on* the ball? Why does his 'will to do' fail him at the critical moment?

What is the stimulus that constitutes an apparently irresistible temptation to him to take his eyes off the ball, in spite of his desire to follow his teacher's instructions and in spite of his 'will to do'?

To answer these questions we shall have to take them in their connexion with each other, for the answers are as closely related to one another as the questions are themselves.

To take the first question.

When the golfer starts to make his stroke, he brings to the act the same habitual use of his mechanisms that he brings to all his activities, and since for such an essential part of the recognized golfing technique as 'keeping his eyes on the ball' the mechanisms concerned with the control of his eyes fail to function as he desires, we are justified in concluding that this habitual use is misdirected. This fact is practically admitted by the instructor when he attributes his pupil's failure to make a good stroke to his failure to keep his eyes on the ball.*

To the question why he continues to take his eyes off the ball, in spite of his intention to follow his teacher's instructions and in spite of his 'will to do', the answer is that in everything he does he is a confirmed 'end-gainer'. His habit is to work directly for his ends on the 'trial and error' plan without giving due consideration to the means whereby those ends should be gained. In the present instance there can be no doubt that the particular end he has in view is to make a good stroke, which means that the moment he begins to play he starts to work for that end directly, without considering what manner of use of his mechanisms generally would be the best for the making of a good stroke. The result is that he makes the stroke according to his habitual use, and as this habitual use is misdirected and includes the wrong use of his eyes, he takes his eyes off the ball and makes a bad stroke. It is clear that as long as he is dominated by his habit of end-gaining, he will react to the stimulus to 'make a good stroke' by the same misdirected use of himself, and will continue to take his eyes off the ball.

This process is repeated every time he tries to make a good stroke, with the result that his failures far outnumber his successes, and he becomes more or less disturbed emotion-

---

*I admit, of course, that a wrong use of other parts might have a more direct bearing upon the golfer's problem, but for the purpose of illustration I have chosen the wrong use of the eyes, because the experts are unanimously agreed (as unanimously as experts ever are) that failure to keep the eyes on the ball is one of the most common and persistent hindrances to the making of a good stroke.

ally,* as always happens when people find themselves more
often wrong than not, without knowing the reason why. And
the more he finds himself unable to carry out his teacher's
instructions with anything like the necessary degree of cer-
tainty for him to get any pleasure out of the game, the worse
this emotional condition becomes. The immediate effect is that
he tries harder than ever to make a good stroke, falls into the
old wrong way of using his mechanisms, and again takes his
eyes off the ball.

Now one would suppose that repeated experience of failure
would of itself lead him to set to work on a different principle,
but my teaching experience goes to shew that in this respect the
golfer's method of procedure is in no way different from that of
other people who use themselves wrongly, and who are trying,
without success, to correct a defect. Strange as it may seem, I
have always found that a pupil who uses himself wrongly will
continue to do so in all his activities, even after the wrong use has
been pointed out to him, and he has learned by experience that
persistence in this wrong use is the cause of his failure.

This apparent anomaly can be explained, and in explaining
it I hope to shew not only what is at the bottom of the golfer's
difficulty, but also of the difficulty which so many people
experience when, with the best 'will' in the world, they find
themselves unable to put right something which they know to
be wrong with themselves.

The habitual use of his mechanisms which the golfer brings
to all his activities, including golf, has always been accompanied by certain sensory experiences (feelings) which, from their
lifelong association with this habitual use, have become
familiar to him. Further, from their very familiarity, they have
come to '*feel right*', and so he derives considerable satisfaction
from repeating them. When, therefore, he attempts to 'make a
good stroke', he brings to the act of swinging his club his faulty

*Unsuccessful effort in any sphere of activity tends to produce emotional
disturbance which is not conducive to healthy recreation. For this reason
alone the golfer whose efforts to carry out his teacher's instructions are
mostly unsuccessful should reconsider his plan of campaign.

habitual use, including the taking of his eyes off the ball, because the sensory experiences associated with this use are familiar and 'feel right'.

On the other hand, the use of his mechanisms which would involve his keeping his eyes *on* the ball during the act of making a stroke would be a use entirely contrary to his habitual use and associated with *sensory experiences which, being unfamiliar, would 'feel wrong' to him*; it may therefore be said that he receives no sensory stimulus in that direction. Any sensory stimulus he receives is in the direction of repeating the familiar sensory experiences which accompany his faulty use, and this carries the day over any so-called 'mental' stimulus arising from his 'will to do'. In other words, the lure of the familiar proves too strong for him and keeps him tied down to the habitual use of himself which *feels right*.

This is not surprising, seeing that the golfer's desire to employ his habitual use at all costs in gaining his end, on account of the familiar sensory experiences that go with it, is an instinctive desire which mankind has inherited and continued to develop all through the ages. *The desire to feel right in the gaining of his end* is therefore his primary desire, in comparison with which his desire to make a good stroke is new and undeveloped, and exerts only a secondary influence. This is proved by the fact that although he starts out with the desire to make a good stroke, his desire to repeat sensory experiences that 'feel right' acts as a stimulus to him to use himself in the habitual way which is associated with these experiences, although it is this very manner of use that prevents him from satisfying his newer desire to make a good stroke.

The desire to carry out his teacher's instructions to keep his eyes on the ball is a still newer desire, and consequently suffers in intensity as compared with the other two. Moreover, it stands even less chance of being carried out, firstly, because the stimulus which gives rise to it does not come from within, like the others, but from without, ie, from the teacher, and secondly, because the instruction is framed with the purpose of correcting something wrong with the pupil's use, ie, the use of the eyes, and so is bound to come at once into conflict with the pupil's desire to employ his faulty habitual use which, as we have just explained, is the dominating influence in whatever he tries to do. The conflict between these two desires is therefore bound to be an unequal one, and his desire to carry out his teacher's instructions goes by the board.*

It is the dominating influence of his desire to gain his end by means of a use of his mechanisms which *feels* right, but is in fact wrong for the purpose, that explains not only why he *continues* to take his eyes off the ball and so to fail in his stroke, but also why, in spite of this repeated experience of failure, he does not give up 'end-gaining' and set to work in a different way.

Now that we have seen the faulty principle which underlies the golfer's efforts to obey his teacher's instructions, we will go on to examine the principle on which these instructions are based.

The instruction to the pupil to 'keep his eyes on the ball' shews that the teacher recognizes that the mechanisms concerned with the control of the pupil's eyes do not function as they should, but when, in order to meet this difficulty, he simply tells his pupil to 'keep his eyes on the ball', he also shews that he does not connect the faulty functioning of the eyes with misdirection of the use of the mechanisms throughout the organism. This means that in his diagnosis and treatment he is not considering his pupil's organism as a working unity in which the working of any of the parts is affected by the working of the whole. To this extent, therefore, his diagnosis may be said to be incomplete and his scope of usefulness as adviser to his pupil limited.

Evidence of misdirection of use in human activity is to be found on all sides, and our real interest in the golfer's difficulty

---

*It must be remembered that the greater his desire to obey his teacher, the greater will be his incentive to increase the intensity of his efforts, and it is practically certain that in his attempts to translate this desire into action, he will automatically increase the already undue muscle tension which he habitually employs for the act, thus lessening still further his chances of making a successful stroke.   Cf. page 62, second note.

is that it is a difficulty not confined to golf, but experienced by all who are trying, without success, to correct defects which hamper them in their various activities, or to perform a certain act satisfactorily.

Misdirection of use is to be found in the person who takes up a pen to write and proceeds at once to stiffen the fingers unduly, to make movements of the arm which should be made by the fingers, and even to make facial contortions; in the physical culturist whose performance of certain movements of the arms or legs, or of both, is associated with harmful and unnecessary depression of the larynx and with undue tension of the musculature of the thorax; in the person who in reading or singing or talking 'sucks' a breath in through the mouth at the beginning of each sentence, though in the ordinary way, in walking or standing, he would breathe through the nostrils; in the athlete, amateur or professional, who, whenever he makes a special effort, employs excessive tension in the muscles of the neck and pulls the head back unduly.

In all these cases, which might be elaborated indefinitely, it will be found that the use of the mechanisms concerned with the movement required is often far removed from that which would best serve the purpose.

This all goes to shew that in every form of activity the use of the mechanisms which comes into operation will be satisfactory or unsatisfactory according to whether our direction of that use is satisfactory or otherwise. Where the direction is satisfactory, satisfactory use of the mechanisms of the organism as a working unity will be ensured, involving a satisfactory use of the different parts, such as the arms, wrists, hands, legs, feet and eyes. It follows that where there is misdirection, this satisfactory use of the mechanisms is not at our command. This is exactly the position of the golfer who cannot keep his eyes on the ball when he desires.

Let us now see how the golfer's difficulty would be dealt with by a teacher who adhered to the idea of the unity of the organism, and so based his teaching practice on what I call the 'means-whereby' principle, ie, the principle of a reasoning consideration of the causes of the conditions present, and an indirect instead of a direct procedure on the part of the person endeavouring to gain the desired end.*

First he would diagnose the golfer's failure to make a good stroke as due to misdirection of the habitual use of the mechanisms, and not primarily to any specific defect such as an inability to keep the eyes on the ball. He would recognize that the inability to keep the eyes on the ball was merely a symptom of this misdirection, and could not by any stretch of imagination be said to be the cause of his failure to make a good stroke. He would observe that immediately his pupil started to make his stroke, he brought into play the same faulty use which he habitually employed for all his activities, and so himself brought about the very thing he wanted to prevent, the taking of his eyes off the ball. He would see that his pupil's difficulty was to a great extent caused by his own 'wrong doing'.

A teacher who made a diagnosis on these lines would understand that the difficulty could not be met by any such purely specific instruction as telling his pupil to keep his eyes on the ball, for he would recognize that any 'will power' exerted by a pupil whose use of himself was misdirected would be exerted in the wrong direction,† so that the harder he tried

---

*Compare *Constructive Conscious Control of the Individual*, p. 10 note.

†Not long ago a professor brought a friend to watch a lesson given to one of his students in whose progress they were both interested on account of her attainments. 'You should have no difficulty with this pupil,' he said, 'because she is so willing and anxious to help you'. 'Yes,' I replied, 'that is one of the curses of the "will to do".' His companion held up her hands in horror at this, exclaiming, 'Surely, even if it's wrong, it's better to exert the "will to do" than not.' This gave me the chance to point out that the 'something wrong' meant that there was a wrong direction somewhere, so that what she was really urging was that the addition of the stimulus of the 'will to do' would be beneficial, even though it involved an increased projection of energy in the wrong direction. It is not the degree of 'willing' or 'trying', but the way in which the energy is directed, that is going to make the 'willing' or 'trying' effective.

to carry out such an instruction and the more he 'willed' himself to succeed, the more his use would be misdirected and the more likely he would be to take his eyes off the ball. From this he would conclude that he must find some way of teaching his pupil to stop the misdirection of his use, and as he observed that the misdirection began the moment the pupil tried to gain his end and make a good stroke, obviously his first step would be to get the pupil to stop 'trying to make a good stroke'. He would explain that any immediate reaction to the stimulus to make a good stroke would always be by means of his wrong habitual use, but that if he prevented this immediate reaction, he would at the same time be preventing the misdirection of his use that went with it and was *the* obstacle to the gaining of his end. He would impress upon him that of all the activities that go to the making of a good stroke, *this act of prevention was the primary activity*, since by the inhibition of the misdirected habitual use the way would be left clear for the teacher to build up in his pupil that new direction of the use of his mechanisms, which would constitute the means whereby he would in time be able to keep his eyes on the ball, and thus make a good stroke.

Now if we are to understand the 'means-whereby' principle on which the teacher who adheres to the idea of unity in the working of the human organism will base his teaching method, we must recognize that the attainment of any desired end, or the performance of any act such as the making of a golf stroke, involves the direction and performance of a connected series of preliminary acts by means of the mechanisms of the organism, and that therefore, if the use of the mechanisms is to be directed so as to result in the satisfactory attainment of the desired end, the directions for this use must be projected in a connected series to correspond with the connected series of preliminary acts. If at any point in the series the chain of directions is broken and use misdirected, all the succeeding acts of the series will go wrong, and the end will not be attained in the way desired (for instance, the golfer will not make a *good stroke). In most people today the direction of the use of their mechanisms is not reasoned out, but instinctive, and in cases where this instinctive direction leads to faulty use, the connected series of acts preliminary to the gaining of any end will be brought about by a series of instinctive directions operating through faulty use of the mechanisms, so that a series of faulty acts will be the result.* *

These facts must be taken into account by the teacher who is using the 'means-whereby' principle to build up a new direction of the pupil's use. He will recognize in his practice that these preliminary acts, though means, are also ends but not isolated ends, inasmuch as they form a co-ordinated series of acts to be carried out 'all together, one after the other'.† He will impress upon his pupil that to maintain the unity that is involved in this connected series of acts, he will have to continue to project the directions necessary to the performance of the first act of the series *concurrently* with projecting the directions necessary to the performance of the second, and so on throughout the series until all the preliminary acts have been performed in their connected sequence and the ultimate end in this way secured.

It may be asked what, exactly, is the technique for putting the 'means-whereby' principle into practice in building up a new and satisfactory direction of use.

It is impossible to put down here more than a bare outline of this technique, because the sensory experiences which come to the pupil in the process of acquiring a new direction of his use cannot be conveyed by the written or spoken word, any more than the most detailed account that a professional golfer can give of his own sensory experiences when making a drive will enable his pupil to reproduce those experiences. But I would

---

*See *Constructive Conscious Control of the Individual*, pp. 264 *et seq.*

†This process is analogous to the firing of a machine gun from an aeroplane, where the machinery is so co-ordinated that each individual shot of the series is timed to pass between the blades of a propeller making 1,500 or more revolutions to the minute.

refer my readers back to Chapter I where I described the experiments which led to my discovering that there is a primary control of the use of the self, which governs the working of all the mechanisms and so renders the control of the complex human organism comparatively simple.

This primary control, called by the late Professor Magnus of Utrecht the 'central control', depends upon a certain use of the head and neck in relation to the use of the rest of the body, and once the pupil has inhibited the instinctive misdirection leading to his faulty habitual use, the teacher must begin the process of building up the new use by giving the pupil the primary direction towards the establishment of this primary control. The pupil will then project this direction whilst the teacher with his hands brings about the corresponding activity, *the combined procedure securing for the pupil the new experience of use which is desired*. This experience, though unfamiliar at first, will become familiar with repetition.

The teacher then gives the secondary direction to the pupil who *must keep the primary direction going*, whilst he projects the secondary direction and whilst the teacher brings about the corresponding activity. This combined procedure again secures for the pupil the new experience of use that is desired, and again this new experience, though unfamiliar at first, will become familiar with repetition.

By this method of procedure the two directions and their corresponding activities become linked together and will remain linked, and if still further directions are required to bring about the desired change in use, the same combined procedure must apply.

As long as teacher and pupil continue to work together on these lines, never deviating in their procedure from the 'means-whereby' principle, they will in time establish in the pupil the desired direction of the use of his mechanisms, and this procedure has only to be repeated until the experiences associated with it have become familiar for the new and satisfactory use to become established in all his activity.

When this stage is reached, it will be found that the

improvement in the pupil's manner of use is associated with an improvement in his standard of functioning, and that undesirable specific symptoms, such as unsatisfactory use of the eyes, have disappeared *in the process*. This means that the golfer will be able to keep his eyes on the ball when he wishes to do so, for new and reliable 'lines of communication' will have been laid down, which ensures that what he 'wills' to do he ultimately does; his 'will-to-do', in short, will be effective.

THE END-GAINER'S DIFFICULTIES WITH THE MEANS-WHEREBY

The objection has often been made that this process would prove too lengthy for the ordinary person. I admit, of course, that *if* some way could be found of inducing the golfer who cannot keep his eyes on the ball to inhibit his desire to make a good stroke without going through the process of changing his faulty use of himself, he would then be able to keep his eyes on the ball and make his stroke successfully.* But in all the years that I have been teaching pupils whose use of themselves is wrong, I have never yet found any of them able to inhibit the desire to gain an end directly until this unsatisfactory use has been changed. Even when they have been made aware of the means whereby they can make the change from unsatisfactory to satisfactory use and functioning throughout the organism and by this means overcome indirectly their specific defects, their desire to gain their end directly is so strong that they are very seldom able to profit by these 'means-whereby' either to the satisfaction of themselves or of their teachers.

This leads me to the point I wish above all to emphasize, namely, that *when a person has reached a given stage of unsatisfactory use and functioning, his habit of 'end-gaining' will prove to be the impeding factor in all his attempts to profit by any teaching method whatsoever*. Ordinary teaching methods, in whatever sphere, cannot deal with this impeding

*This applies equally to any other difficulties a golfer may experience in his play.

factor, indeed, they tend actually to encourage 'end-gaining'.*
The instruction given to the golfer of our illustration to keep
his eyes on the ball is typical of the kind of specific instruction
given by teachers generally for the purpose of eradicating
specific defects in their pupils, and, as we have seen in his case,
this instruction was a stimulus to him to try harder than ever to
gain his end, and so to misdirect his efforts worse than ever.†

This habit of 'end-gaining' is so ingrained that it will create
a serious difficulty even where the teaching method is based on
the 'means-whereby' principle, and the difficulty can only be
overcome if both teacher and pupil at every step in their
combined procedure, even the simplest, adhere strictly to the
working principle I have set down, namely, that in a series of
acts which have been thought out as the means whereby a
given end can be satisfactorily gained, the primary act must
not be considered as an end in itself, but must be directed and
carried out and *then continued* as the preliminary means of
carrying out the secondary act, and so on.

My daily teaching experience has shewn me that the great
stumbling-block in the way of the pupil's co-operation in this
plan is his idea that as long as he grasps 'intellectually' the
principle underlying the 'means-whereby' procedure and
subscribes to it fully in theory, he will have little difficulty in
working to it practically'.‡ It is true that a pupil may start out
with an 'intellectual' conception of what is required for the

---

*This criticism applies to methods employed by teachers of all sports and
games, of physical culture, eurythmics, dancing, singing, etc.

†Even supposing it were possible to restore *at once* to a pupil satisfactory
direction of his use and functioning throughout the organism, the pupil's
habit of end-gaining would still persist in acts in which he was practised in
employing his old familiar use, as, for instance, in making a golf stroke, so
that the moment he attempted to make the stroke by his new unfamiliar
direction of use, he would bring into play his old habitual misdirection of
use, take his eyes off the ball and make a bad stroke.

‡This is a belief that will probably be shared by my readers and is quite
understandable, since it is difficult for anyone who has not had the actual
experience of working on the 'means-whereby' principle to realize what
unity of 'physical' and 'mental' processes means in practice.

'means-whereby' procedure, but in my experience I have found that the moment the idea of performing any act in that procedure comes to him, his habit of 'end-gaining' causes him to *try to 'do' the act in the habitual way that feels right*, and this in spite of the fact that I have repeatedly demonstrated to him that the sensory appreciation upon which he is depending to 'know' whether his means are right or not is deceiving him, so that what he feels is the right use of himself in gaining his end is in fact wrong.

In the case of such a pupil, working on the 'means- whereby' principle means working against a habit of life, and difficult as it is to work to a principle against any habit of life (as anyone who tries it will find out), the difficulty is enormously increased when it comes to working contrary to the habit of 'end-gaining', for this habit is so closely bound up with faulty habits of use which feel right, that to give it up means giving up the lifelong familiar habits of use that go with it, and employing in its stead a new use which feels wrong.

I therefore claim that if any habit so confirmed as that of 'end-gaining' is to be changed and not merely transferred, it is essential that the pupil should be given the experience, at first in the simplest activities,

(1) *of receiving a stimulus to gain a certain end and refusing to react to it*, thereby inhibiting the unsatisfactory habits of use associated with his habitual reaction;

(2) *of projecting the directions for the new and more satisfactory use* in their proper sequence, primary, secondary, etc, 'all together, one after the other', as already explained, *whilst the teacher at the same time with his hands makes him familiar with the new sensory experiences** associated with this new use.

By this procedure a gradual improvement will be brought about in the pupil's sensory appreciation, so that he will become more and more aware of faults in his habitual manner of using himself; correspondingly, as with this increasing

*I must again impress upon the reader that these new sensory experiences will at first feel wrong.

awareness the manner of his use of himself improves, his sensory appreciation will further improve and in time constitute a standard within the self by means of which he will become increasingly aware both of faults and of improvement, not only in the manner of his use but also in the standard of his functioning generally.* And since it is by means of the use of the self that he reacts to all stimuli, it is clear that together with the improvement in the manner of the use of his mechanisms and in the adjustment of the different parts of his organism, there will also come about an improvement in his manner of reacting to stimuli in every sphere of activity. This improvement will necessarily include an improvement in his manner of reacting to the stimulus to gain a certain end, shewing that it is possible, by working to the principle involved in the 'means-whereby' procedure, to strike at the very roots of the habit of end-gaining which is so deeply embedded in our make-up.

It is obvious that a procedure that makes for the control of the manner of reacting to stimuli must make for the control of habit generally, and for this reason the technique which I have outlined for the building up of a conscious direction of the use of the self should make an appeal to all those who are interested in education in its widest sense.

*For instance, with the improvement in his use he will become aware of an increase in the expansion and contraction of the thorax, ie, of the degree of thoracic mobility. Reliability of the sensory register is essential to all who would make permanent changes from unsatisfactory to satisfactory conditions of functioning.

CHAPTER IV

The Stutterer

I will take for my second illustration the case of a man with an impediment in his speech who was sent to me for advice and help. He told me that he had taken lessons from specialists who treated speech defects, and had done his best to carry out their instructions and to practise their exercises. He had always had special difficulty with sounds which called for the use of the tongue and lips, particularly with the consonants T and D, but although he had been more or less successful in doing the exercises themselves, his stutter was as bad as ever in ordinary conversation, especially when he was hurried or excited.

As is my custom with a new pupil, I noted specially the way he walked into my room and sat down in a chair, and it was obvious to me that his general use of himself was more than usually harmful. When he spoke, I also noticed a wrong use of his tongue and lips and certain defects in the use of his head and neck, involving undue depression of the larynx and undue tension of the face and neck muscles. I then pointed out to him that his stutter was not an isolated symptom of wrong use confined to the organs of speech, but that it was associated with other symptoms of wrong use and functioning in other parts of his organism.

As he doubted this, I went on to explain that I had been able to demonstrate to every stutterer who had come to me for help that he 'stuttered' with many other different parts of his body besides his tongue and lips. 'Usually,' I said, 'these other defects remain unobserved or ignored until they reach the point where the wrong functioning manifests itself in some form of so-called "physical" or "mental" disorder. In your case, your stutter interferes with your work and hinders intercourse with your fellows, and so you have not been able to ignore it, but this may well turn out to be a blessing in disguise if it is the means of making you aware, before too late, of the other more serious defects which I have pointed out to you, and which will tend, as time goes on, to become more and more exaggerated.' I assured him that my long years of practical experience in dealing with the difficulties and idiosyncrasies of people who stutter had convinced me that stuttering was one of the most interesting specific symptoms of a general cause, namely, misdirection of the use of the psycho-physical mechanisms, and I did not wish to take him as a pupil, unless he was prepared to work with me on the basis of correcting this misdirection of use generally, as the primary step in remedying his defects in speech. I could promise him, however, that if he decided to come to me and I was successful in making certain changes for the better in his manner of using his mechanisms, a change for the better would also come about in the functioning of his organism, and his stuttering would tend to disappear in the process. He saw the point and decided to take lessons.

Now in my experience stuttering, like the golfer's tendency to take his eyes off the ball, is due to habitual misdirection of the use of the mechanisms, so that the remedying of the defect in both cases presents fundamentally the same problem. Like the golfer, the stutterer needs to have this habitual misdirection of his use changed to a more satisfactory direction, and the new and improved use, associated with this change in direction, has to be built up and sufficiently stabilized in him before he will be able to employ it practically as a means of overcoming his particular difficulties in speaking.

In the case of this pupil, therefore, I began by pointing out to him various outstanding symptoms of his wrong habitual use, one of the most marked of these being the undue amount of muscle tension that he was in the habit of employing throughout his organism whenever he tried to speak. This extreme muscle tension was an impeding factor in the functioning of his mechanisms generally, and rendered impossible a satisfactory use of his tongue and lips, and the more he tried by any special effort of 'will' to speak without stuttering, the more certain he was to increase the already undue muscle tension and so to defeat his own end.

The reason for this, I explained to him, was that he did not start to speak until he had brought about the amount of tension which was associated with his habitual use and which caused him to *feel that he could speak*; ie, he would decide that the moment had come for him to speak only when his *feeling* told him that he was using his mechanisms to the best advantage, and this moment, in the last analysis, was when his sensory appreciation (the only guide he had as to the amount of muscle tension necessary) registered to him as 'right' the amount of tension which he habitually employed in speaking and which was therefore familiar to him.

Unfortunately, the familiar amount of tension that 'felt right' to him was the unnecessary amount associated with the wrong habitual use of his mechanisms of which his stuttering was a symptom, and I therefore urged him to recognize from the beginning that the 'feeling', upon which he was relying to tell him when his use was right for speaking, was untrustworthy as a register of muscle tension, and that he must not depend upon it for guidance in his attempts to speak. How, I asked him, could he expect to judge by his feeling the amount of tension he should employ in speaking, when he was unfamiliar with the sensory experience of speaking with the due amount? Obviously, he could not 'know' a sensation he had never experienced, and as sensory experience cannot be conveyed by the spoken word, no amount of telling on my part could convey to him the unfamiliar sensory experience of speaking with less tension and without stuttering. The only way to convince him that he could speak with a less amount of muscle tension would be to give him this unfamiliar experience.

To this end I adopted a procedure based upon the same principle as the procedure employed to the end of giving the golfer the experience of keeping his eyes on the ball, my aim being to give my pupil, first, the experience of employing a conscious direction of a new and improved use of his mechanisms generally, and, secondly, the experience of *continuing to employ this conscious direction whilst using* the mechanisms concerned with the act of speaking in the manner best suited for the purpose.

I began by giving him

(1) the directions for the inhibition of the wrong habitual use of his mechanisms associated with the excessive muscle tension;

(2) the directions for the employment of the primary control leading to a new and improved use which would be associated with a due amount of muscle tension.

I then asked him to project these directions whilst I with my hands gave him the new sensory experiences of use corresponding to these directions, in order that the trustworthiness of his sensory appreciation in relation to the use of his mechanisms might be gradually restored, and that by this means he might in time acquire a register of the due amount of tension required for speaking, as distinct from the undue amount of tension associated with his stuttering.

I continued this procedure, until I had repeated for him the new sensory experiences of use often enough to justify me in allowing him to attempt to employ his new 'means-whereby' for speaking and for saying the words and consonants that caused him special difficulty.

It is impossible in the space at my command to put down all the details of the variations of the teacher's art that were employed to bring my pupil to this point, for a teacher's technique naturally varies in detail according to the particular needs and difficulties of each pupil. Those of my readers, however, who have followed the account of the difficulties I encountered when I first attempted to employ the new 'means-whereby' in my reciting, will be able to realize the kind of difficulty we were faced with all along, when I say that my pupil was a confirmed 'end-gainer'.

At the beginning of this new stage in our work together I reminded him how his progress up to this point had been hampered by his habit of end-gaining and of 'trying to be right', and I warned him that unless he succeeded in side-stepping it, he would have little chance of applying his new 'means-whereby' to his difficulties in speaking, for if, at the critical moment of starting to say a difficult word, he still went directly for his end and tried to say the word in the way that 'felt right' to him, he would be bound to revert to his old habitual use in speaking and so stutter.

Events proved how difficult it was for my pupil to take practical heed of this warning. I would repeatedly urge him, whenever I gave him a sound or word to pronounce, always to inhibit his old habitual response to my request by refusing to attempt to pronounce the sound or word until he had taken time to think out and employ the new directions for the use which he had decided upon as best for his purpose. He would agree to do this, but as soon as I asked him to pronounce some sound or word, he would fail to inhibit his response to the stimulus of my voice, and forgetting all about the new directions he had been asked to employ, he would immediately try to repeat the sound, with the result that he was at once dominated by his old habits of use associated with the extreme muscle tension that *felt right* to him, and so stuttered as badly as ever.* In short, his very desire to 'be right in gaining his end' defeated the end.

In every stutterer of whom I have had experience this habit of reacting too quickly to stimuli is always associated with sensory untrustworthiness, undue muscle tension and misdirection of energy, but in this pupil's case the habit of going directly for his end, and of trying to 'feel right' in doing it, had been positively cultivated in him by the methods employed by his previous teachers in trying to 'cure' his stutter.†

---

*In order that the reader should not think this difficulty was peculiar to this pupil, I wish to state that I have had similar experiences with all my pupils. How could it be otherwise when 'end-gaining' is a universal habit?

†See Chapter III, page 67, second note.

It would appear that the 'end-gaining' principle underlies every one of the exercises given by teachers who, whether by orthodox or unorthodox methods, deal with stuttering as a specific defect, and I will take as an example the exercises that had been given to my pupil to meet his special difficulty in pronouncing words beginning with T or D.

His former teachers had recognized that the use of his tongue and lips was unsatisfactory for the purpose of pronouncing these consonants, and in order to overcome the difficulty had instructed him to practise certain exercises involving the use of these specific parts in saying T or D.

Now this procedure could only aggravate the difficulty, for the idea of trying to say T or D acted as an incentive to the pupil to employ the habitual use of himself associated with the wrong use of his tongue and lips. As long as this wrong habitual use remained unchanged, this association persisted and he had little chance of getting rid of this incentive, so that to ask him under these conditions to practise saying T and D as a remedy for his stuttering was tantamount to giving him an added incentive to stutter.

This was borne out by what I observed when he shewed me how he had been practising these exercises. I watched him closely and saw that as soon as he started to do them, he at once made an undue amount of tension generally, continued to increase the tension of the muscles of the lips, cheeks and tongue, and tried to say T and D before his tongue had taken up the best position for the purpose. This attempt was as bound to result in failure as would be the attempt of a motorist to change gears before the clutch has done its work in getting the cogs into the position in which they will mesh. It was evident that he had been trying in all his practice in the past to gain his end without being in command of the means whereby this end could be successfully gained, and the fact that the majority of these attempts had been unsuccessful had brought him to a state of lack of confidence in himself, which added considerably to the difficulty of breaking his 'end-gaining' habit.

As far as I am aware, all methods of 'curing' stuttering, however they may differ in detail, are based on the same 'end-gaining' principle. The adviser will select some symptom or symptoms as the cause of his pupil's stuttering and will give him specific instructions or exercises to help him.

I am well aware that it has proved possible by such methods to stop people from stuttering, but I would question the common assumption that because this is so, a genuine 'cure' has been effected. For in cases where it is claimed that a stutter has been 'cured', there is usually something peculiar or hesitating about the manner of speaking, and those concerned do not seem in the least perturbed that the harmful conditions of undue muscle tension, misdirection of energy and untrustworthiness of sensory appreciation, present in the case when the 'cure' was begun, are still in evidence now that what is considered a successful 'cure' has been brought about.

No method of 'cure' can be accepted as effective or scientific, if, in the process of removing certain selected symptoms, other symptoms have been left untouched and if new, unwished-for symptoms have appeared.* If this test is applied to a stutterer after he has been 'cured' by such methods, it will be found too often that the original defects of undue muscular tension, misdirection of energy and untrustworthiness of sensory appreciation have been increased in the process of the 'cure'.†

I admit that these defects may not bring about a recurrence

---

*As Dr Dewey writes in his Introduction to *Constructive Conscious Control of the Individual*, 'the essence of scientific method does not consist in taking consequences in gross; it consists precisely in the means by which consequences are followed up in detail. It consists in the processes by which the causes that are used to explain the consequences or effects, can be concretely followed up to shew that they actually produce these consequences and no others.'

†As an example of this, I will quote a statement made to me by an intending pupil at his preliminary interview. He told me, among other things, that he had cured himself of stammering and I asked him how he had done it. He replied that he had been a very bad stammerer, but that one day

of the stutter, but even so, they are almost certain to lead to the further development of other undesirable symptoms which constantly remain unrecognized. This invariably happens when defects and diseases are 'cured' by specific methods, and explains why, in spite of the immense number of 'cures' recorded, the troubles in the human organism would seem to be increasing and calling for more and more 'cures'.

It is important to remember that there is a working balance in the use of all the parts of the organism, and that for this reason the use of the specific part (or parts) in any activity can influence the use of the other parts, and vice versa. Under instinctive direction this working balance becomes habitual and 'feels right', and the point at which the influence of the use of any part will make itself felt will vary and the influence of the particular use be strong or weak according to the nature of the stimulus of the end activity desired. If a defect is recognized in the use of a part, and an attempt is made to correct this defect by changing the use of the part without bringing about at the same time a corresponding change in the use of the other parts, the habitual working balance in the use of the whole will be disturbed. Unless, therefore, the person attempting to make a change in the use of a specific part has an understanding of what is required to bring about at the same time a correspond-ing change in the use of the other parts which will make for a satisfactory working balance and therefore be complementary

he was forced to run to the top of a long flight of stairs to deliver an important message, and found to his surprise that after this experience he was able to speak without stammering, and he had continued to be able to do so. Most people, of course, would look upon this as a 'cure', but I could not, because I saw that his use of himself generally was still very bad, and when I said so, he admitted that he suffered from other troubles which, in my opinion, amounted to 'stuttering' in other parts of his organism. The fact is, the experience to which he attributed his freedom from stammering had not changed his unsatisfactory conditions of use to those satisfactory conditions which are not found in association with stammering. Consequently, similar experience was just as liable to cause a recurrence at any time of the vocal stammering, and as his unsatisfactory manner of use was still present, he had a predisposition to develop other troubles.

to the new use that he is trying to bring about at one point, one
of two things is bound to happen:

either, (1) *the stimulus of the desire to gain his end, by
means of the old use associated with the habitual working
balance which 'feels right', will be so strong that it will
dominate the stimulus to cultivate a new and improved use
of a certain part associated with an unfamiliar working
balance which 'feels wrong';*

or, (2) *if the change in the use of a part is made in the face of
impeding factors in the use of the other parts (as happens in
any specific method of treatment employed to correct a
defect in a part), the working balance between the use of
that part and the use of all the other parts will be so thrown
out of gear that the use of the other parts will be adversely
affected in their turn, and new defects in the use of these
parts developed.*

After my pupil had shewn me the exercises he had been told to
do, I explained to him that in practising them he had been
indulging in his old wrong habits of general use of himself, and
thereby actually *cultivating* the wrong habits of use of his
tongue and lips which had made him stutter. I impressed upon
him once more that if he wished ever to be confident of saying
T and D and words in which these consonants occur without
stuttering, *he must refuse to respond to any stimulus either
from within or without to say T or D*; in other words,
whenever the idea of saying T or D came to him, he must
inhibit his desire to try and say it correctly, until he had learned
what use of his tongue and lips was required in his case for
saying T or D without stuttering, and until he could put into
practice the necessary directions for this new use of his tongue
and lips *whilst continuing to give the directions for the
primary control of the new and improved use of himself
generally.*

He understood the reason for this, but his attempts at co-
operating with me proved more or less unsuccessful for some
time. Over and over again I got him to the point where the
use of his tongue and lips in association with his general use

was such that I knew he could pronounce T and D without the undue muscle tension that made him stutter, but when at this point I asked him to repeat one of the sounds, he would either

(1) forget to inhibit his old response, change back to his old conditions of use and increase the tension to the point when he *felt* that he could say T or D, try to say it in this way and stutter, or

(2) on the occasions when he remembered to inhibit his old response and to employ the new 'means-whereby' for saying T and D without stuttering, he would make no attempt to repeat the sound.

In both these cases he was actuated by the same motive. He associated the act of speaking, especially the pronunciation of consonants that were difficult for him, with a given amount of muscle tension, and as I have already shewn, he had come to believe that it was impossible for him to speak until he *felt* this undue amount of tension. This explains why he made no attempt to speak until he had deliberately brought about the familiar but excessive tension which caused him to stutter. In this way he simply reinforced the old sensory experiences of undue muscle tension already associated with his habitual use, and with his habit of trying to *feel right* in gaining his end.

To deal with this difficulty I made a point of giving my pupil day after day the experience of receiving a stimulus to gain a certain end and of remembering to refuse to gain that end, since this refusal meant that at one fell swoop he inhibited all the wrong habits of use associated with his habitual way of gaining that end.* In proportion as he was successful in inhibiting his immediate response to any stimulus, he became able to defeat his desire to gain his ends in the way that felt right to him, and *as long as he continued this inhibition*, I on my side was able to repeat for him, until they became familiar, the new sensory experiences associated with an improved

---

*Cf. Chapter I, pp. 40ff; Chapter III, pp. 68ff.

general use of his mechanisms, including the right use of his tongue and lips. By continuing to co-operate with me on these lines, he gradually acquired sufficient experience in the direction of this new use to be able to employ it successfully as the 'means-whereby' of pronouncing the consonants which had caused him special difficulty.

But, more important than this, my pupil in the course of this procedure had learned that if he inhibited his immediate instinctive reaction to any stimulus to 'do', he could prevent the misdirection of his use and the associated undue muscle tension which had been the marked feature of all his reactions to stimuli, and which had hampered him not only in his speaking but in all his activities, both 'physical' and 'mental', and if he chose to apply this principle to his activities in other spheres, he would have at his command a means of controlling the nature of his reaction to stimuli, that is, of acquiring a control of what is called 'conscious behaviour'.*

*The following is of interest in this connexion. One of my pupils has just told me that before he came to me for lessons he used to have uncontrollable fits of temper, but that since having the work he has no trouble in that way, and that all his family notice the change. He asked me to explain how it was that what he looked upon as a 'nervous' or 'mental' symptom could be affected by the kind of work I was doing with him. In reply I asked him how other people knew when he had lost his temper, and he answered that they would know by the tone of his voice, the expression of his face, the look in his eyes, or by his gestures and excited manner generally. I then asked him how these reactions could be possible except through the use of what he thought of as his 'physical' self. For instance, the voice must be used if we are to judge its tone, there must be use of the eyes if they are to flash, of the muscles of the face for change of expression, and, for excitability to be manifested, the whole of the mechanisms of use must be stimulated into undue activity and muscle tension.

Change the manner of use and you change the conditions throughout the organism; the old reaction associated with the old manner of use and the old conditions cannot therefore take place, for the means are no longer there. In other words, the old habitual reflex activity has been changed and will not recur. If loss of control can be manifested only by means of the use of ourselves, it follows that a conscious direction of an improving use will bring us for the first time within striking distance of a conscious control of human reaction or behaviour.

Certain features of this pupil's case occur with practically every pupil.

During the earlier stages of a pupil's lessons when the use of his mechanisms is still unsatisfactory, I have constantly found that he fails to inhibit the old instinctive direction of his use, with the result that his directions for the new use do not become operative. Before I can get a chance to help him, he proceeds to gain his end in accordance with his habitual wrong use, and it is practically impossible under these circumstances to stop him from gaining his end in this way.

On the other hand, when he has learned at a later stage in his lessons to inhibit the instinctive direction of his use and the directions for the new use have become operative, so that I am enabled to give him the corresponding sensory experiences, I have found that although he now has at his command the best conditions possible for gaining his end, he will not make any attempt to gain it. He cannot believe that the end can be gained with these improved conditions present; they 'feel so wrong', as he puts it, that he instinctively refuses to employ them.

When this difficulty arises, it is necessary for me to give him the actual experience of gaining his end by what he feels is a wrong use of his mechanisms, and when I have succeeded in doing this, he invariably remarks how much easier the new way is than the old way, and how much less effort it requires. Yet in spite of this admission, the actual experience of gaining his end in this new way has to be repeated for him again and again before the improved use 'feels right' to him, and before he gains the necessary confidence in employing it.

The lesson to be learned from all this is that since our particular way of reacting to stimuli is in accordance with our familiar habits of use, the incentive to try to gain any given end is inextricably bound up with this familiar use. This explains why, if a pupil's familiar use is changed to one that is unfamiliar and therefore unassociated with his habitual way of reacting to stimuli, he has little or no incentive to gain that given end. As long as the conditions of use and the associated

feeling are wrong in a person, the incentive to gain a given end
by the familiar wrong use appears to be almost irresistible, but
when these conditions have been changed to conditions which
are best for the purpose of gaining the end, there seems to be
practically no incentive to gain it.

This is not surprising, for when a person's sensory appreciation of his use is wrong and his belief as to what he can or
cannot do is based on what he feels, gaining an end by a use
that is unfamiliar means for him taking a plunge in the dark.
Even when I have explained to a pupil why this difficulty has
arisen in his case, and he understands the reason for it
'intellectually', he will need, more often than not, considerable
encouragement and practical assistance in order to be enabled
to make the experience of gaining a given end by means of a
use that is new and unfamiliar to him. Once this has been done
for him, however, he becomes conscious of a new experience
that he is desirous to repeat, and repetition of this experience
in time convinces him that his previous beliefs and judgments
in this connexion were wrong. As a result there gradually
develops in him an incentive to employ the new use, and this
becomes at last far stronger than the incentive to employ the
old use, for its development is the outcome of a reasoned
procedure which he finds he can consciously direct and control
with a confidence he has never before experienced.

One of the most remarkable of man's characteristics is his
capacity for becoming used to conditions of almost any kind,
whether good or bad, both in the self and in the environment,
and once he has become used to such conditions they seem to
him both right and natural. This capacity is a boon when it
enables him to adapt himself to conditions which are desirable, but it may prove a great danger when the conditions are
undesirable. When his sensory appreciation is untrustworthy,
it is possible for him to become so familiar with seriously
harmful conditions of misuse of himself that these malcon-
ditions will feel right and comfortable.

My teaching experience has shewn me that the worse these
conditions are in a pupil and the longer they have been in

existence, the more familiar and right they feel to him and the harder it is to teach him how to overcome them, no matter how much he may wish to do so. In other words, his ability to learn a new and more satisfactory use of himself is, as a rule, in inverse ratio to the degree of misuse present in his organism and the duration of these harmful conditions.

This point must be understood and taken into practical consideration by anyone forming a plan of procedure for improving the use and functioning of the mechanisms throughout the organism as a means of eradicating defects, peculiarities and bad habits.

Towards the end of his lessons my pupil asked me why it should be so much more difficult to overcome the habit of stuttering than the habit of over-smoking. He then went on to tell me that at one time he had been an inveterate smoker, but realizing that the habit was getting too much of a hold on him, he had decided he must give it up. He had first tried the plan of reducing the number of cigarettes he smoked per day, but as he found that he could not keep within the prescribed limit, he had decided that the only way for him to succeed in breaking his habit was to give up smoking altogether. He put this decision into practice and had become a non-smoker. He now wanted to know why his efforts to overcome his stuttering had not been equally successful.

I pointed out to him that the two habits presented very different problems.

The smoker can abstain from smoking without interrupting the necessary activities of his daily life, and as the temptation to smoke to excess results, as every chain-smoker knows, from the fact that each pipe, cigar or cigarette smoked acts as a stimulus to the smoking of another, every time he abstains from smoking he is breaking a link in the chain.

The stutterer, on the other hand, cannot abstain from speaking because his daily intercourse with his fellows depends on it. Every time he speaks, therefore, he is thrown into the way of temptation to indulge in his familiar wrong habits of use of his vocal organs, tongue and lips, and so to stutter. The stimulus to speak is one that he cannot evade in the way a smoker can evade the stimulus to smoke if he so wills it, so that the habit of stuttering calls for a much more fundamental form of control.

Satisfactory control of the act of speaking demands a satisfactory standard of the general use of the mechanisms, since the satisfactory use of the tongue and lips and the required standard of control of the respiratory and vocal organs depend upon this satisfactory general use. This being so, the unsatisfactory general use of the mechanisms which, as we have seen, is present in every stutterer, constitutes a formidable obstacle in the way of mastering his habit.

The situation is very different for the smoker, for the act of smoking does not demand any such high standard of use of the mechanisms, and although unsatisfactory conditions of use are frequently present in his case, the influence which they exercise in preventing him from overcoming his particular habit is small in comparison.

Still another element enters into the case. The habit which the smoker is trying to overcome is one which he has himself developed in the process of satisfying a desire. The stutterer, on the other hand, is dealing with a habit which has not been developed in the process of satisfying a desire, but which has gradually grown to become part of the use of the mechanisms which he habitually employs for all the activities of his daily life. This explains why the smoking habit is relatively superficial and in this degree easier to overcome, and why my pupil had been able *by himself* to solve the problem of his over-smoking, but had not been able to deal with his habit of stuttering without the help of a teacher who understood how to give him the means whereby he could *himself* command that satisfactory use of his mechanisms generally which includes the correct use of the tongue, lips and vocal organs for the act of speaking.

I would emphasize here that the process of eradicating any such defect as stuttering by these means makes the greatest demands on the time, patience and skill of both teacher and pupil, since as we have seen, it calls for

(1) the inhibition of the instinctive direction of energy associated with familiar sensory experiences of wrong habitual use, and

(2) the building up in its place of a conscious direction of energy through the repetition of unfamiliar sensory experiences associated with new and satisfactory use.

This process of directing energy out of familiar into new and unfamiliar paths, as a means of changing the manner of reacting to stimuli, implies of necessity an ever-increasing ability on the part of both teacher and pupil to 'pass from the known to the unknown';* it is therefore a process which is true to the principle involved in all human growth and development.

Since this chapter was written, I have received a letter from this pupil, and with his permission I am quoting the following extracts from it, as they are of interest in relation to the development of sensory awareness of an improvement in use:

> I hope that you have not construed my prolonged silence to mean that I have lost interest in you or in your work. Quite the contrary is the case. I am interested in little else . . . I feel quite sanguine about the possibility of making considerable progress again if I can come this year. I am optimistic enough to believe that I am almost ripe for some real new experiences . . . I have now come to the point that when I feel my back working I also feel my jaws relax. I really believe that I have been using my jaw muscles to keep myself erect! I am really beginning to appreciate how little I have used my tongue and lips in my speech, in fact, I have scarcely used them at all. It is this great improvement in my sensory appreciation that gives me such hope for the future.

*The late Mr Joseph Rowntree after one of his lessons described my work as 'reasoning from the known to the unknown, the known being the wrong and the unknown being the right'.

CHAPTER V

Diagnosis and Medical Training

For many years medical men have been sending their patients to me, because they know that I am experienced in examining conditions of use and in estimating the influence of these conditions upon functioning. I would say at once that I do not receive these cases as patients, but as pupils, inasmuch as I am not interested in disease or defects apart from their association with harmful conditions of use and functioning.

Some of the cases have been previously diagnosed and treated for such widely differing troubles as angina pectoris, epilepsy, locomotor ataxia, rheumatoid arthritis, sciatica, infantile paralysis, asthma, neuritis, so-called nervous and mental troubles, constipation, voice and throat trouble, flatfoot and stuttering, and on examination of each of these cases I have found present unsatisfactory functioning associated with harmful use of the psycho-physical mechanisms.

In other cases the doctors have been unable to find any cause or explanation of the patient's symptoms, which in some instances have been symptoms of so-called mental trouble such as carelessness, depression, lassitude, unreliable memory, inability to give attention to the job in hand, undue excitability and a low standard of accomplishment generally, and, in other instances, symptoms of a more recognizably 'physical' character, such as sleeplessness, indigestion, malnutrition, poor circulation and chilblains. On examination of such cases also I have always found present undesirable conditions of use of the self which have not been recognized, and which have tended to lower the general standard of functioning in the patient.*

*Every medical man has records of cases in which he has been unable to find any specific trouble calling for treatment.

Further, in all cases where I have found harmful conditions of use and functioning in association, I have also found that the sensory appreciation (that is, the knowledge which comes to us through the sensory mechanisms as to the manner of our use of ourselves) is not to be depended upon, with the result that the sensory direction of use in all activity is faulty, manifesting itself in bad habits in the everyday acts of walking, sitting, standing, eating, talking, playing games, thinking and reasoning, etc.

My experience in all these cases has brought home to me the close relationship which exists between the manner of use of the mechanisms and the standard of functioning, for where I have found unsatisfactory use of the mechanisms, the functional trouble associated with it has included interference with the respiratory and circulatory systems, dropping of the abdominal viscera, sluggishness of various organs, together with undue and perverted pressures, contractions and rigidities throughout the organism, all of which tend to lower the standard of resistance to disease.

On the other hand, in cases where disease has been previously diagnosed in any of the organs or systems, I have found that the faulty functioning which this implies is always associated with an unsatisfactory manner of use throughout the organism.

This goes to shew that an unsatisfactory manner of use, by interfering with general functioning, constitutes a predisposing cause of disorder and disease, and that anyone who makes a diagnosis and prescribes treatment, without finding out how much of the trouble present has arisen from this interference and how much from other causes, is leaving untouched a predisposing cause of disorder and disease.

For this reason I make the following claim:

(1) No diagnosis of a case can be said to be complete, unless the medical adviser gives consideration to the influence exerted upon the patient, not only by the immediate cause of the trouble (say, a germ invader), but also by the interference with functioning which is always

associated with *habitual* wrong use of the mechanisms and helps to lower the patient's resistance to the point where the germ invader gets its opportunity.

(2) Since the medical curriculum does not include training in the knowledge of how to direct the use of the human mechanisms, the medical man does not bring to his diagnosis an understanding of 'use' in the sense I have defined, and so does not recognize the relationship between misdirection of use and that unsatisfactory standard of functioning which is always found in association with disease; any deductions he may make, therefore, will be based on incomplete premises, and the value of his work limited both in the field of prevention and of cure.

(3) A training in the satisfactory direction of the use of his own mechanisms is essential to the medical man's personal equipment; for in the course of this training he would be gaining a knowledge which would enable him to judge the manner of use present in the patient, detect any misdirection of use, and, where this exists, determine its relation to any symptoms of unsatisfactory functioning present.

In support of this claim I will take as an illustration the orthodox practice of making tests for the purposes of diagnosis, and I choose 'tests' because the result of any test of conditions in a patient is bound to be more or less influenced by the manner of that patient's habitual use of his mechanisms, and if this influence is not taken into consideration, any diagnosis based on the test must to that extent be incomplete.

To prove this we have only to make a test of functioning on a person in whom there are present certain unsatisfactory conditions of use, and make the same test again on that same person after the conditions of use have been changed for the better, and the result of the second test will be found to differ from that of the first; in the majority of cases, indeed, we shall find a marked difference between the two.

An instance in point occurs to me. I was called by a specialist to a case for consultation, and when I went into the room he was testing the patient's chest and lungs with a stethoscope. I realized at once that here was one of the worst cases of wrong use I had ever seen, with the associated contraction and immobility of the thorax, depression of the larynx, tendency to hold the breath in the ordinary acts of life, and harmful stoop. His manner of use was impeding his respiratory processes and · circulation and the action of his heart, influencing adversely even his pulse and blood pressure. When the specialist had finished, he asked me to listen so that I could get some idea of the patient's respiratory difficulties from the medical standpoint. I did so, and after noting the result with him, I pointed out the symptoms of wrong use I had observed, and suggested that if he would allow me to make even a slight change in these conditions of use, and then made the same test again whilst I maintained the changed conditions in the patient, the stethoscope would register an entirely different result. He agreed, I made certain changes,* maintained them whilst the second test was made, and the specialist on using the stethoscope found that what I had predicted had taken place. He sent the patient to me with ultimately satisfactory results.

I will now go further and try to shew that the medical man is limited, even more in preventive work than in the field of 'cure', because he does not recognize the influence of satisfactory use in the maintenance of a desirable standard of general functioning, and so, when he comes to make his diagnosis, he does not possess the knowledge that would enable him to distinguish between satisfactory and unsatisfactory conditions of use in any case he is examining.

Take the case of a child whose parents take him to a doctor purely as a preventive measure. The child shews no symptoms of illness, but the parents want to make sure that there are no harmful tendencies latent which, if allowed to develop

*I am prepared to demonstrate that, given a reasonable subject, a temporary change to more satisfactory conditions of use can be brought about in a short space of time, although the patient is bound to fall back almost immediately into his wrong habitual use.

unchecked, might lead later on to illness or defect of some kind or another. The doctor examines the child, and finds no symptoms or tendencies which in his opinion call for attention or treatment. He therefore gives the child a clean bill of health.

In appraising the value of this opinion, we must again take into account that the medical curriculum does not include any training that would enable a medical man to employ a satisfactory direction of his own use in the acts of daily life, or to teach his patients to do the same. It is therefore not unreasonable to assume that the doctor of our illustration, when examining the child, does not know what unsatisfactory conditions of use are present, and that if they were present, he would not be likely to recognize them or to estimate their influence upon functioning. He cannot be expected to look out for something, however potent a factor this may be in the development of tendencies to disease and disorder, when he is not even aware of its existence. Consequently, his study of the child's general conditions cannot be said to be complete, for he may give the child a clean bill of health and yet leave unrecognized and unchecked in him conditions of use which, if allowed to develop, may lead in time to the lowering of the child's standard of functioning and resistance to disease.

As an example of a diagnosis based upon a recognition of the close relationship between use and functioning I will cite the following case. On December 12, 1923, a medical man wrote to me as follows:

> I have just read your book *Man's Supreme Inheritance* as a result of Dr Peter Macdonald's remarks at the BMA Meeting. I am a medical man and have had to take a rest on account of angina pectoris, and the principles underlying your work appeal to me as being really sound, so much so that I would like to put them into practice in my own case. I am 61, and up to two months ago I was engaged in active practice . . . If you can help me I should be glad of a reply.

An interview was arranged, and when Dr X came to see me,

I proceeded in my usual way to make an examination of the conditions of use present. After this examination I told him that I found that his use of himself was most unsatisfactory, shewing a high degree of misuse and maladjustment associated with a dangerous lowering of the standard of functioning of the respiratory, circulatory and digestive systems. This combination of harmful conditions is one which I have always found present in a marked degree in cases of angina pectoris, and would, in my experience, be sufficient in itself to account for the distressing sensations* experienced by the patient.

This being my diagnosis, I explained to Dr X that my method of dealing with his case would be to try and change his unsatisfactory conditions of use to those more desirable conditions which are only found present in association with satisfactory functioning. From the first, Dr X was particularly interested in my method of diagnosis, and this interest increased as he recognized that during the process of building up a new and more satisfactory use which he employed more or less in his daily life, the symptoms which gave rise to the diagnosis of angina, and which had incapacitated him from work and from playing golf became less and less in evidence in proportion to the change and improvement in the conditions throughout his organism, and so far disappeared that he became free from pain and able once more to work and to play golf.† He described the work I was doing as the 'first clinical physiology for the human being', and realizing that my method of diagnosis differed fundamentally from that employed in orthodox medical practice, he urged me to write on the subject in order to put my findings before the medical profession.

In what follows I shall make an attempt to carry out his suggestion, and I think I cannot do better than base the

*A medical friend tells me that these sensations, as described to a doctor, constitute the only available evidence upon which a case can be diagnosed as one of angina pectoris.

†July 10, 1931. I saw this pupil a few days ago and the good work still goes on. F.M.A.

comments I have to make on an address that was delivered by
Lord Dawson of Penn at the House of Commons on February
24, 1926,* because I am assured by my medical friends that
the views which Lord Dawson there expressed, as to the
efficacy of medical training as a preparation for the successful
diagnosis of disease, can be taken to represent current medical
opinion on this subject.

My comments will of necessity involve some criticism of
medical training, for a lack in the medical curriculum has been
brought home to me in my capacity as an educator, but in view
of Lord Dawson's statement at the opening of his address that
'of criticism itself the profession made no complaint whatever', and seeing that I am able to offer a technique which I am
convinced from my experience would make good this lack, I
have the best of reasons for believing that members of the
profession will give this criticism their consideration.

On the subject of *Diagnosis and the Medical Curriculum*
Lord Dawson said that

A necessary preliminary to treatment was a knowledge of
disease . . . its causes and its diagnosis. To attempt to treat
disease without knowing what is wrong with the body as a
whole (not with a part only) was admittedly an act of folly,
and to gain such knowledge there must be carefully
organized training . . . There should be no recognition of a
man as an independent practitioner until he had had those
years of training, and had studied the nature of disease and
its diagnosis . . . And the training should be the same for all.
In this matter there could not be the least compromise . . .
Whatever a man's views on navigation might be, whatever
his genius, he was not allowed to assume control of a ship
until he had passed the tests for navigators. Why should less
protection be afforded to the human ship sailing on the sea
of life? . . . Everyone was now trying to get control of
disease more early, in its more curable stages, and hence

*The Report of Lord Dawson's address from which I am quoting will be
found in *The Lancet* of March 6, 1926.

diagnosis was of supreme importance.*

Let me begin with Lord Dawson's statement that 'a necessary preliminary to treatment was a knowledge of disease — its causes and its diagnosis.'

It is obvious that once we are aware of the cause of disease, we have some chance of dealing successfully with it, and that there would be less tendency for parts of the organism to become diseased if the functioning of these parts were satisfactory. The connexion between disease and wrong functioning should be generally recognized and it should also be recognized that where specific symptoms of disease have been diagnosed, *the associated wrong functioning is always associated in its turn with undesirable use of the mechanisms of the organism as a whole.* This association has been borne in upon me by my teaching experience, which has taught me that *in the process* of improving the use and functioning of the organism *as a whole* specific symptoms of disease tend to disappear or to be eradicated.

I therefore fully agree with Lord Dawson that 'to attempt to treat disease without knowing what is wrong with the body as a whole (not with a part only)' is 'admittedly an act of folly'. But when he implies that the 'carefully organized' medical training of today does give the student this essential knowledge, I join issue with him on the ground that there is nothing in medical training which would enable a member of the medical profession

(1) to detect and diagnose that wrong *habitual* use of the mechanisms which is associated with wrong functioning and therefore with symptoms of disease, and

(2) to follow up his diagnosis by a process of correcting wrong habitual use and building up in its place a satisfactory use of the mechanisms, a process which, because it is always accompanied by improvement in the standard of functioning, invariably tends to the

*The italics are mine. F.M.A.

re-establishing of conditions associated with health.

Now it is clear that such a method of diagnosis and treatment differs fundamentally in principle from orthodox medical methods, whereby definite local symptoms are traced back to specific disorders which are diagnosed as the cause of the trouble and then treated specifically. Suppose, for instance, a general practitioner finds symptoms which he diagnoses as due to trouble in some part, or parts, such as the heart, liver, eye, lung or any other, he will either treat the trouble in the specific part or parts himself, or else send the patient on to a specialist who will proceed to prescribe treatment specially adapted to meet the trouble in that specific part or parts.

I admit, of course, that by this method specific symptoms may be and often are eliminated, but since

(1) specific symptoms are never found apart from wrong functioning,

(2) the wrong functioning associated with such symptoms is always, in my experience, associated with wrong use of the mechanisms of the organism,

(3) by such methods nothing will have been done to improve this wrong use,

conditions will be left within the organism which, if allowed to develop unchecked, will tend to lower the standard of functioning generally, and it will then be only a matter of time before the trouble — either the original disorder, or, as frequently happens, some more serious trouble — will manifest itself.

I submit, therefore, that no person who has not been trained, firstly, to detect the wrong use which is associated with wrong functioning, and secondly, to employ a technique evolved to the end of correcting this wrong use, can diagnose 'what is wrong with the body as a whole' or treat the body as a working unity, and that since the study of medicine does not include any such training, and no such technique has been employed in the treatment of disease, the methods of training championed by Lord Dawson cannot give medical students the help they need to enable them to diagnose 'what is wrong with the body as a whole'.

I cannot accept Lord Dawson's analogy between medical training and the training for navigation. How can it be maintained that medical training includes a knowledge of the 'human ship sailing on the sea of life', when the medical student is taught nothing about the use of the mechanisms (either in his own case or in that of his patients) upon which the control of the 'human ship' depends? Whatever training a navigator may have received in the management and control of his ship, he would be helpless without a reliable compass to determine his direction. If by chance he took a wrong course and on investigation found that his compass had gone wrong, he would not attempt to proceed until he had seen to it that his compass was put right.

This is where the analogy between the training for medicine and the training for navigation seems to me to break down. For sensory appreciation is to the 'human ship sailing on the sea of life' what the compass and other such guides are to the navigator's ship; it is the only guide we have to shew us if in our daily activities we are directing the use of our mechanisms to the best advantage. But the medical man, in his work of navigating the 'human ship', does not recognize that sensory appreciation is frequently at fault, and so he proceeds on his course attempting to guide the 'human ship' without first seeing to it that his compass is reliable. It has never been recognized in medical practice that sensory appreciation, the human compass, has become more and more unreliable with the advance of civilization, and that in proportion there has come about a growing misdirection of the use of the human organism.

Man has been faced with no greater problem than this. For, as we have seen, the nature of a man's reactions to stimuli in general is in accordance with the manner of the use of his mechanisms, and since use cannot be satisfactory without a reliable sensory direction of that use, his reactions to stimuli will be unsatisfactory in proportion as his sensory appreciation is untrustworthy.

I believe that most of us today are more or less in need of help in cultivating that higher standard of sensory appreciation of use which leads to a more satisfactory control of reaction, and this applies no less to the medical man than to the layman. This is borne out by the practical experience of both, who have constant proof in themselves of unreliability of the sensory mechanisms resulting in such unsatisfactory forms of reaction to stimuli as faulty observation and a low standard of awareness in general. For instance, in cases where it is necessary for several medical men to be consulted, there is too often a wide variance of opinion among them, and we have only to read medical evidence in the law courts to find striking examples of differing diagnoses among men who have all undergone the same 'carefully organized' medical training. Many medical men, indeed, deplore the fact that in spite of medical training,* members of the profession frequently do not possess the equipment upon which successful diagnosis primarily depends.

Everyone will agree that for accuracy and efficiency in diagnosis the medical man needs to possess not only a high standard of sensory observation and awareness, but also the ability to link phenomena together, to form sound judgments and to take a wide outlook, especially in the presence of unfamiliar conditions. To attain these qualities he needs reliability of the sensory mechanisms concerned with the direction of use of the whole organism in daily activity, and the ability to control instinctive reactions to stimuli, especially reactions to the stimulus of the unfamiliar.

It is my belief that this need can be met by the employment of

*It will be remembered that the late Sir James Mackenzie, as a result of researches made by him and his collaborators at the St Andrews Institute of Clinical Research, found that seventy per cent of human ailments are not yet identified. I have also before me, as I write, an article entitled 'Doctor's Vain Guesses', in which the Medical Correspondent of *The Times* discusses the protest made by the Ministry of Health against the institution of record cards 'on the ground that our knowledge is as yet insufficient to make general records valuable', and in striking confirmation of this view he cites the findings of the late Sir James Mackenzie to which I have referred.

a technique for the building-up of a conscious direction of the use of the mechanisms, for I have found in my practical experience with pupils that in the process of learning to acquire a conscious in the place of an instinctive direction of their use, there comes about a corresponding improvement in their standard of functioning throughout the organism, and in the nature of their reactions generally.

The explanation of this lies in the nature of the process itself. For the fact that the pupil receives from the hands of the teacher the actual sensory experience of the new use which he is consciously directing, ensures for that pupil a gradual cultivation of sensory trustworthiness and awarenesss, whilst the second fact that the pupil is not able to employ in his daily activities the new use associated with this unfamiliar sensory experience, until he has consciously inhibited his instinctive desire to employ his familiar habitual use, means that he is gradually developing a reasoning control of his instinctive reactions to stimuli, especially his reactions to the stimulus of the unfamiliar.

Although this technique is concerned more with education than with treatment, it is one which, as I have tried to shew, should be incorporated with medical training, for if this were done, and the medical student taught how to consciously direct the use of his own mechanisms, he would be developing within himself a satisfactory standard in his sensory appreciation which would stand him in good stead in diagnosing defects in others. But further, in his treatment of these defects, he would no longer be satisfied to employ purely specific treatment for dealing with specific symptoms, for he would have learned from his personal experience that by a process of restoring and maintaining in activity a reasoning direction of the use of his mechanisms, a satisfactory standard in the functioning of the organs and systems is likewise restored and maintained. For reasons of expediency, of course, he might still be forced in certain circumstances and crises to treat a specific trouble directly, but working on the principle of the indivisible unity of the human organism and equipped with the technique based upon it, he could be both what I will call a 'generalist'* applying this knowledge practically to the requirements of his patient's case, and also an educator, in that he would be called upon to teach his patient to direct and maintain a satisfactory use of himself in all his activities. Basing his teaching and treatment on the principle of unity, he could hardly fail to recognize the connexion between use and functioning which this implies. He would therefore relate any specific defects or symptoms, which he found present in specific organs or parts, to interference in the interworking of the mechanisms generally, and his method of dealing with such specific trouble would be to correct his patient's wrong habitual use of his mechanisms as the means of correcting the specific wrong functioning associated with particular symptoms or defects; at the same time he would teach his patients how to direct and maintain a new and improved use which, *if employed in all his activities*, would be the means of preventing the recurrence of the old or the development of further defects.

In order to illustrate how this has worked out in my experience I will give three examples, the first of which is particularly pertinent here, since most medical men must have had cases of patients who have experienced in the convalescent stage difficulties similar to those which I describe.

EXAMPLE I

The first is the case of a lady who had a long and serious illness during which she was ordered to remain in bed for several months, and she underwent a long course of treatment. The time came when she was told that she could begin to get up and try to walk a few steps at a time, and that as the muscles gradually became stronger, she would in time be able to walk properly. She followed this advice, and after a few months she was able to get about a little with the aid of a stick, but only with great difficulty and fatigue, as acute pain developed in her

*The word 'generalist' has been coined for me by my friend Dr Peter Macdonald of York.

knees and ankles, which became worse when she walked. The doctor, however, encouraged her to go on trying to walk more, 'a little more every day'. But this she found she could not do, and as time went on, instead of being able to walk further with less difficulty, the reverse was the case, until her condition became such that if she walked at all on one day, she was obliged to rest upon the next. This condition grew gradually worse, but what caused her real anxiety was that certain symptoms of her original illness gave evidence of returning, and she was then persuaded by a friend who knew my work to consult me.

When she came to see me, I recognized that the manner of her habitual use of herself was most harmful, and that in everything she was doing she was using herself in such a way as to bring about harmful pressures. The results of her work with me proved this to be so, for as I was able to bring about an improvement in her manner of use and to teach her how to direct and maintain it consciously, these pressures gradually decreased. At the time of coming to me she was only able to have six lessons as she was going away to the sea, but after having been away for a short time she wrote to me that she was doing her best to carry on the work, and that she was now able to walk the length of the Parade with only occasional intervals of rest. By the end of the summer she could walk up and down stairs with some degree of ease, and had managed three miles at a stretch. On returning to town in the autumn, she began regular work with me and as an improvement in her use was brought about, the pains gradually disappeared and by the end of that winter she was living a normal life and walking with ease and comfort. In the last four years she has had no return of the original symptoms, in spite of the fact that she now includes gardening among her activities.

EXAMPLE II
This pupil had been treated for months by a well-known specialist in Boston, because he suffered from severe pains in the lower part of his back, particularly when walking, and his

pulse and blood pressure were abnormal. He had been given remedial exercises, and an abdominal belt to wear as a support. As this treatment was not successful, an operation had been suggested, but he had not agreed to this and had come to London to consult another specialist. This specialist after making an examination sent him to me as he believed that the change that I could bring about in his general condition would relieve the pressure and muscular rigidity, which, in his opinion, was the cause of the pain.

When he came to see me, I asked him to perform some of his remedial exercises for me, and as I watched him doing them, it was obvious to me that the wrong manner of use which was present in him had been exaggerated by his practice of these exercises. He was employing an undue amount of tension for the simplest acts, and when he walked, his tension was increased to such an extent that it was not surprising that walking even a short distance caused him intense pain.

I decided that this was a case that could be helped by my work, and I proceeded to shew him how to prevent the wrong manner of using himself which he had been taught in these exercises, and at the same time I gave him directions for the new manner of use which, as I brought it about for him, would relieve the pressure and strain of the lower spinal articulations, which was responsible for his pain and which had been aggravated by his practice of the remedial exercises.

After a few days' lessons the pupil felt relief, and he soon decided that he could dispense with the support he had been wearing. At the end of the second week he was able to take short walks without pain, and after an eight weeks' course of lessons, his medical adviser agreed with me that he was in a fit condition to return to America. Ten months later he returned to England and called to see me. He told me that in the interval he had done his best to keep up what I had taught him and that he had been free from the old pain and discomfort, had not needed to wear any support, and that his doctor, after a recent examination, had said that his pulse and blood pressure were now normal.

EXAMPLE III

My third example is that of a young woman who wished to be enrolled as a student of an Institution for the Training of Teachers, but on being medically examined, had been told that her condition of health was such that she would not be able to stand the strain involved in the work of training. The doctor who examined her said that he could not diagnose anything definitely wrong that would warrant his prescribing medical treatment; what she needed was outdoor life and freedom from duties which called for effort of any kind. The Principal of the Institution, who was acquainted with my work, brought her to see me, when I found that the manner of her general use of herself would account for the lack of stamina that the medical diagnosis indicated. The upper part of her chest was unduly depressed and her thoracic capacity and mobility reduced to the minimum, seriously affecting her circulation. She also told me that she suffered from chilblains on the hands and feet, and the slightest exertion caused fatigue.

I told her that I could enable her to take the Training Course provided that she came to me for lessons at the same time, and the Principal, understanding the reason for this, made this arrangement possible. She started her training and at the same time a course of lessons with me, and the improvement in her manner of use which gradually resulted so improved her standard of general functioning, that she has been able to meet the demands of her training without interruption, and now, at the completion of her course, is able to take up her work as a teacher.

I have been asked whether the technique I advocate is applicable to cases of people who are anxious, not so much to remedy a so-called physical defect, but to overcome or change what they think of as 'mental' or 'nervous' troubles, including bad habits of all kinds,* as they realize that as long as they

*By these I mean such habits as absent-mindedness, forgetfulness, lack of awareness and observation, undue excitability, twitching, plucking at

cannot control these, they are not getting the best out of themselves. My answer is that the fact that these people are unable to make a change within themselves, which they have reasoned out would be a desirable change, shews that their reaction to the stimulus to gain this end is an unsatisfactory reaction, and that this brings their case at once into line with that of the golfer who cannot keep his eyes on the ball when he wishes to, and of the stutterer who cannot speak as he desires.

I will say at once that of course no one could give a general definition of a satisfactory reaction which would meet the particular circumstances of every case, but we shall surely all agree that in cases where people wish to improve themselves, or to make changes which they consider will be for their good, or to overcome defects and bad habits, their reaction may be considered satisfactory when they succeed in doing what they have reasoned out is the right thing for them to do.

This should make it clear that we are not here concerned with fixed standards of value as to what constitutes right or wrong in any particular case. Such standards are relative and more or less individual, for a man's beliefs and acts are largely the outcome of his upbringing and circumstances, and therefore should not be judged by any fixed standard of right and wrong. Acts which are held to be right by one race and at one period are often condemned by other people or at other periods. Circumstances and conditions play a great part in the question, and each case has to be judged on its own merits.

But where the use of the self is concerned, there is a standard which can generally be accepted, for it can be demonstrated that a certain manner of use of the mechanisms is found in association with a certain satisfactory standard of functioning and with conditions of health and general well-being. We are surely justified in considering a manner of use that is associated with such desirable conditions to be 'natural' or 'right' under all circumstances. But this is not a fixed standard of 'right' in the accepted meaning of the word, for this manner of

fingers, inability to sit still, nail-biting, over-sensitiveness, uncontrollable temper, inattention, etc.

use being based upon a primary control of the mechanisms of the organism is one that can be applied and adapted to meet all circumstances, and its 'rightness' may therefore be said to be relative to these circumstances. Further, the experiences involved in acquiring a knowledge of such 'right' and 'natural'* use of the self gives a person a criterion of judgment to go by, and also an understanding of relative values, for in this process he is constantly brought up against situations in which, after receiving a stimulus, he has to decide what manner of use is the best to employ in reacting to it, and also to judge which of the directions for this manner of use is primary, which secondary, and so on. The standard of relative values that he thus acquires is one that will stand him in good stead in reacting to the stimuli of modern life, in which conditions change so constantly that they cannot be adequately met by any external standard or fixed code as to what is right or wrong. Seeing that the self is the instrument of all his activities, it follows that a valid criterion relating to the use of this self will be a criterion that is valid in relation to all his activities, both so-called 'mental' and 'physical'.

It is the lack of a valid criterion as to what constitutes right use in the sense of 'right for the purpose' that renders people unable to carry out their resolutions and to make certain changes for the better in themselves and in their conduct and attitude towards others. Like the golfer and the stutterer, they want to make a change, but bring into play for the purpose the only use of themselves they know, that use, with its associated habits, which we have called throughout this book the 'habitual' use of the self, and the fact that, when using themselves in this habitual way they do not succeed in doing what they have reasoned out is the right thing to do, indicates that their habitual use is misdirected and faulty for the purpose. As long as they have no other criterion to go by but that of the familiar *feeling* of their wrong habitual use, the use they employ will be wrong for the purpose, and their reaction

*By 'natural' I do not mean usual; indeed, 'natural' in this connexion is, as a rule, the very opposite of usual.

to the stimulus to make the desired change will be their instinctive reaction and therefore directed along the old wrong channel.

To meet this difficulty I would apply to their case the technique which I advocate for the building up of a conscious direction of use, for its employment demands that instinctive reaction be inhibited and superseded by reasoning processes. I have found that *in this process* of acquiring a conscious direction of use my pupils gradually develop a higher standard of sensory awareness or appreciation of what they are doing in the use of themselves, so that when it comes to carrying out a course of activity they have decided upon, they possess a criterion *within themselves* which will enable them to judge whether the use they are employing is right or not for the purpose. This will constitute a criterion of self-criticism where impressions conveyed through feeling, and leading to further experience, are concerned.

I wish, however, to emphasize here the importance of inhibition in this process, for on account of the habit of end-gaining which is practically universal, such difficulties as we have indicated cannot be permanently overcome unless inhibition is allied to the process of reasoning out the right 'means-whereby' and acquiring a higher standard of sensory direction. The reader will remember how, in my own case, my failure to *continue to inhibit*, due to the habit of end-gaining, was *the* obstacle to my employing the new 'means-whereby' in reciting, although I had reached the point where I could command these new 'means-whereby' in ordinary speaking and knew by experience that they were 'right' for my purpose. I have also shewn how the golfer and stutterer of my illustrations, though constantly warned that the habit of end-gaining would be the greatest difficulty they would have to contend against in making the changes in themselves that they desired, were still unable, when the moment came to gain their particular end, to resist the stimulus to gain that end immediately, which meant that they did not continue to inhibit their habitual reaction whilst projecting the directions for the new use, and so reacted by reverting to the wrong habitual use which 'felt right'.

In both these cases the habit of end-gaining led them into doing the wrong thing, the golfer with the use of his eyes, the stutterer with the use of his tongue, and this in spite of their desire to make certain changes for the better in the use of these organs, and in spite of their having learned how to direct the use of their mechanisms generally in such a way as to make these particular changes possible.

For this reason, all those who wish to change something in themselves must learn to make it a principle of life to inhibit their immediate reaction to any stimulus to gain a desired end, and, in order to give themselves the opportunity of refusing to fall back upon the familiar sensory experiences of their old habitual use in order to gain it, *they must continue this inhibition* whilst they employ the new direction of their use. By adhering to this principle they will find that this conscious direction of their use will gradually come to be associated with a sensory criterion upon which they can rely as a more accurate register of impressions.

All my experience goes to shew that in cases where untrustworthiness of sensory appreciation has led to a general misdirection of the use of the mechanisms and to unsatisfactory conditions of functioning, a particular stimulus may start up a sensory process which registers a reaction which is quite different from the reaction which has actually taken place.

This is a fact that can be demonstrated, and in view of the admittedly unsatisfactory adjustment of human beings to the demands of modern civilization, the most serious symptom of which is, in my opinion, the growing untrustworthiness of the sensory processes, it is of special interest to me to find that Sir Arthur Eddington, in his Lecture on 'Science and Religion',* issued the following warning:

*See Reprint *Science and Religion. A Symposium.* (Gerald Howe Ltd, London.)

I have been laying great stress on *experience*; in this I am following the dictates of modern physics. But I do not wish to imply that every experience is to be taken at face value. There is such a thing as illusion and we must try not to be deceived. In any attempt to go deeply into the meaning of religious experience we are confronted by the difficult problem of how to detect and eliminate illusion and self-deception. I recognise that the problem exists, but I must excuse myself from attempting a solution . . . Reasoning is our great ally in the quest for truth. But reasoning can only start from premises; and at the beginning of the argument we must always come back to innate convictions. There are such convictions at the base even of physical science. We are helpless unless we admit also (as perhaps the strongest conviction of all) that we have within us some power of self-criticism to test the validity of our own convictions. The power is not infallible, that is to say, it is not infallible when associated with human frailty . . .

When Sir Arthur Eddington says 'we must try not to be deceived', I would venture to submit that in the light of the experiences I have set down in this book, just 'trying' not to be deceived will not solve the problem he raises. For all 'trying' starts from some personal conviction that in some way we shall be able to do what we are trying to do, and this conviction, like conviction on any other point, is made possible only by virtue of impressions received through the agency of our sensory processes. We must therefore see that the validity of this conviction is dependent upon the nature of the functioning of our sensory make-up. If this is satisfactory, our sensory register of impressions of what we are doing and experiencing in response to the stimulus to 'try' is likely to be a true register; in other words, the reaction we register is likely to be the reaction that is actually taking place. On the other hand, if the functioning of our sensory make-up is un-satisfactory, our register of what is happening in response to the stimulus to 'try' is likely to be deceptive, so that the reaction we register is more than likely to be different from the reaction that has actually taken place.

The reader will remember how in my own case (and this applies equally to the golfer and the stutterer) my 'trying' to do the thing which I believed was the right thing to do was based upon the conviction that if I knew what the right thing was, I should, by trying, in time be able to do it, and it was only after a prolonged experience of constant failure that I was driven to the discovery that I was not doing the thing I believed I was doing when I was 'trying' to do it. This brought me face to face with the fact that my sensory mechanisms were registering impressions which were not the true impressions of what was really happening.

It is therefore clear that the conviction underlying my 'trying', being based upon impressions reaching me through the agency of sensory processes that were untrustworthy, was founded upon a delusion, and to make this conviction, as I did, the premise for reasoning that 'trying' would in time bring about the end I desired was only paving the way to further self-deception.

I make no apology for laying such stress upon this personal experience, for the sensory make-up of mankind is admittedly gradually becoming more and more untrustworthy.* It seems

* We all of us know of occasions when the impression registered within us of some happening has not been an accurate impression of the nature of that happening; how, for instance, our sensory mechanisms can register 'cold' when the thermometer registers otherwise, and how a person will take offence and register a remark as a slight or rebuke, when the speaker intended neither and no one else present registered the remark in that sense. Those who are interested in the subject can find in the newspapers daily proof of the registering of false impressions leading to false judgments in all spheres of life.

See also Introduction to *Constructive Conscious Control of the Individual* where Professor John Dewey writes:

'In all matters that concern the individual self and the conduct of its life, there is a defective and lowered sensory appreciation and judgment, both of ourselves and of our acts which accompanies our wrongly-adjusted psycho-physical mechanisms. It forms our standard of rightness. It influences our every observation, interpretation and judgment. It is the one factor which enters into our every act and thought.'

strange to me that although man has thought it necessary in the course of his development in civilization to cultivate the potentialities of what he calls 'mind', 'soul' and 'body', he has not so far seen the need for maintaining in satisfactory condition the functioning of the sensory processes through which these potentialities manifest themselves. As a result, the functioning of his sensory processes has become so unsatisfactory that the use of his mechanisms is constantly misdirected in his efforts to 'do', and when he 'tries' to put right the results of this misdirection, he has no other criterion for self-criticism to guide him in these attempts but that of the untrustworthy sensory processes which originally led him into error.

We must therefore see the danger of continuing to base our efforts to help ourselves or other people upon beliefs, judgments and convictions which have their source in sensory experiences, without ascertaining whether the mechanisms through which these experiences are conveyed are functioning satisfactorily.

I venture to suggest that the experiences described in this book throw light upon the way in which the functioning of the sensory mechanisms can be so improved that they will afford a more valid criterion for self-criticism. Those who have had the experience of putting into practice the technique I have described for the building up of a conscious direction of their use, have found that the process gives them the opportunity for testing continuously the validity of their sensory observations and impressions of what is taking place, because all the time that they are consciously projecting the directions for the new and improved use, they are obliged to go on *being aware* whether or not they are reverting to the old instinctive misdirection of their use which, associated with sensory untrustworthiness, had led them originally to be deceived in what they were doing with themselves. Further, those who continue to make the principle underlying this procedure their guiding principle in all their activities, find that they are enabled to combine 'thinking in activity' with a new sensory observation of the use of themselves in the process. This means that they are not only aware when their reaction is not what they feel it is or what they desire, but, having at the same time a reasoned knowledge of the means to a better reaction, they are also able consciously to keep in check the old instinctive reaction that has been the obstacle to their doing what they desire.

If a technique which can be proved to do this for an individual were to be made the basis of an educational plan, so that the growing generation could acquire a more valid criterion for self-judgment than is now possible with the prevailing condition of sensory misdirection of use, might not this lead in time to the substitution of reasoning reactions for those instinctive reactions which are manifested as prejudice, racial and otherwise, herd instinct, undue 'self-determination' and rivalry, etc, which, as we all deplore, have so far brought to nought our efforts to realize goodwill to all men and peace upon earth?

APPENDIX

In fulfilment of my promise in the Preface to this book, there follows a reprint of the Open Letter to Intending Students relating to the Training Course for Teachers, and also a reference to the work being done in the little school. The reader will have realized ere now that in the matter of gaining the experience of using ourselves in a new and unfamiliar way in the performance of acts both familiar and unfamiliar, time is 'the essence of the contract'. Experience convinced me that children who came for the ordinary half-hour lesson and attended school outside, or spent the rest of the day without being watched from the point of view of carrying on the work in their daily activities, were not getting a fair chance, and I decided that much better results would accrue if these children could be watched and helped by teachers of my work during their school activities.

The actual simple beginning of the little school at 16 Ashley Place came about in this way. In 1924 a little boy was sent home from India because, although highly intelligent, he was so 'nervous' and excitable that his parents realized he would not be able to cope with the conditions of ordinary school life, and so sent him for lessons. When he arrived, I found that his use of himself was so unusually bad that it was decided that in addition to his private lessons he must stay each day and be helped to employ the new use of himself that he was learning for his reading, writing and other lessons. Parents of other children who were taking lessons at the time then asked that their children also might have this help given to them, and in this way the little school started. Since that time children and young people of all ages who have been taking private lessons have entered the class in order to get experience in applying the principles and procedures involved in the technique to other activities, remaining for periods ranging from a few weeks to several terms. Naturally the nature of the school work done by the members of the class differs according to their different ages and requirements, but it is all based upon the principle inherent in the technique, namely, that the end for which they are working is of minor importance as compared with the way they direct the use of themselves for the gaining of that end.

In this development of the work I have been fortunate in having the co-operation of my brother, Mr Albert Redden Alexander, of Miss Ethel Webb and Miss Irene Tasker, MA, and, later, of Miss E. A. M. Goldie. Miss Tasker had had a wide and varied experience of teaching, both privately and under the Board of Education, before she became a teacher of my technique. She has arranged and conducted the work of the school, since January 1929 with the assistance of Miss Goldie, and the children have had the advantage of help from the whole staff in their private lessons.

We have now had the experience of five months' work of the Training Course for Teachers, and during this first session we have aimed at correlating the individual work of the students, usually done in private lessons, with the group work necessary to give them the experience required for the making of teachers. To this end the students work for some hours daily under the supervision of a teacher, and they devote the rest of the day to the continuance of this class work, helping one another and aiming always at strict adherence to the principle underlying the technique. The results so far attained in this way justify us in believing that at the end of eighteen months' training these students will be able to help in the little school by working with the children under supervision. This would make it possible to give more individual attention to the children, thus enabling them to make greater progress in a given time.

In the Open Letter which follows the reader will find a reference to a scheme for the development of a larger school in the future, together with details of the Training Course.

OPEN LETTER TO INTENDING STUDENTS
OF TRAINING COURSE

16 Ashley Place,
London, S.W.1

For many years past I have devoted much time and thought to the working out of satisfactory means whereby students can be trained to impart the technique set down in my books *Man's Supreme Inheritance* and *Constructive Conscious Control of the Individual*, and in working for this end I have been greatly stimulated by the support given by the members of the medical and other professions who have come to me as pupils. I have hesitated, however, before making definite plans for the practical carrying out of this idea, chiefly,

(1) Because I thought it advisable to be able first to publish the opinion of those most competent to judge whether I am justified in my conviction that I should teach people to carry on my work.

(2) Because the difficulties which I encountered in my attempts to provide possible students with the material for gaining the necessary practical experience in teaching were for a time insurmountable.

(3) Because I wished to be as certain as possible that at the conclusion of the first course of training there would be a demand for teachers of my work.

With regard to (1) I am now able to quote the following educational and medical authorities who have had the opportunity of observing my work and of testing the value of the principle on which it is based, and whose support has finally decided me to start a course for the training of teachers.

Professor John Dewey (Gifford Lecturer, 1929)

The Earl of Lytton, PC, GCSI, GCIE

Sir Lynden Macassey, KBE, KC

Miss E. E. Lawrence (Principal of The Froebel Institute)

Miss Lucy Silcox, Class. Trip. Camb. (Headmistress of St

Felix School, Southwold, from January, 1909, to July,
1926)

A. G. Pite, MC, MA (Headmaster, Weymouth College,
Dorset)

A. J. D. Cameron, MB

Mungo Douglas, MB

Percy Jakins, MD, MRCS

Peter Macdonald, MD

R. G. McGowan, MD, DPH

A. Murdoch, MB

A. Rugg-Gunn, MB, FRCS

From Professor John Dewey (Gifford Lecturer, 1929).
Quotation from Introduction to *Constructive Conscious
Control of the Individual*, pp. xxxi–xxxiii.

'After studying over a period of years Mr Alexander's
method in actual operation, I would stake myself upon the fact
that he has applied to our ideas and beliefs about ourselves and
about our acts exactly the same method of experimentation
and production of new sensory observations, as tests and
means of developing thought, that have been the source of all
progress in the physical sciences; . . . Mr Alexander has found
a method for detecting precisely the correlations between the
two members, physical–mental, of the same whole, and for
creating a new sensory consciousness of new attitudes and
habits. It is a discovery which makes whole all scientific
discoveries, and renders them available, not for our undoing,
but for human use in promoting our constructive growth and
happiness . . . The discovery could not have been made and
the method of procedure perfected except by dealing with
adults who were badly co-ordinated. But the method is not one
of remedy; it is one of constructive education. Its proper field
of application is with the young, with the growing generation,
in order that they may come to possess as early as possible in
life a correct standard of sensory appreciation and self-
judgment. When once a reasonably adequate part of a new
generation has become properly co-ordinated, we shall have

assurance for the first time that men and women in the future will be able to stand on their own feet, equipped with satisfactory psycho-physical equilibrium, to meet with readiness, confidence and happiness instead of with fear, confusion and discontent, the buffetings and contingencies of their surroundings.'

Knebworth House,
Knebworth
March 22nd, 1930

DEAR MR ALEXANDER,

I am delighted to hear that the scheme for the training of students in your work has materialised. You know how anxious I have been that your valuable work for the welfare of mankind should be carried on. The experience you have gained and the technique you have evolved are far too valuable to be lost. There must be thousands who like myself have benefited by your help, but we can do no more than tell others of our good fortune; we cannot pass on to them the benefits we have received. If you can train others to practise your technique and thus found a school for the training of teachers of your work it will be a great service to humanity.

I wish your new venture all success.

Yours sincerely,

LYTTON

27, Abingdon Street,
London, S.W.1
5th April, 1930

DEAR MR ALEXANDER,

It is with the greatest satisfaction that I learn that there is now a definite prospect of arrangements being made for the training of Teachers to acquire and apply your technique and so ensure that your methods will be preserved and perpetuated. It would, in my view, be a calamity if such arrangements were not to be made.

Nothing is required to convince me of the essential value of your work. The beneficial results it has achieved in the cases of persons known to me, who had exhausted all other advice and remedial treatment, are so outstanding as to carry conviction to the mind of anyone who will take the trouble to investigate what you are doing and see what your methods can accomplish.

I am convinced that it is of the greatest public importance that your methods shall be made known and available to the public as widely as possible.

Yours sincerely,
LYNDEN MACASSEY

16th April, 1930

DEAR MR ALEXANDER,

We are delighted to hear that you have decided to train students in the science and art of your educational work.

From our personal experience of your work and our knowledge of the enormous benefits you have given to both children and adults we think it a matter of supreme importance that an attempt should be made to train students in the handing-on of your own technique.

Simple and fundamental as it is, it is at the same time unlike anything we have come across in our educational experience and we feel it impossible to measure the good that will come from it.

Yours sincerely,
ESTHER E. LAWRENCE,
LUCY SILCOX,
A. G. PITE

May 8th, 1930

DEAR MR ALEXANDER,

May we express how pleased we are to learn that you have decided to undertake the training of pupils in the technique which you have discovered, elaborated, and practised for many years and in the important principles on which it is based? As medical men we, more than most people, are conscious of the difficulties involved in the undertaking. We realise that the technique you have to impart, being at one and the same time a very advanced craft and a very subtle philosophy, demands special qualities of mind and a certain natural aptitude of body to practise it with success. We rejoice, therefore, that you are now confident that these difficulties can be overcome. As practitioners of medicine we know also how great is the need for its resources at the present time, when the strain of existence exacts such a toll even on the healthy. We believe, from practical acquaintance of its effects on ourselves and our patients, that it is adequate to meet that need, if only because it teaches that satisfactory use of the self which is the basis of physical and mental happiness.

We wish the extension of your valuable work every success and beg to proffer, in so far as we may, our willing co-operation.

Yours sincerely,

A. J. D. CAMERON, MB
MUNGO DOUGLAS, MB
PERCY JAKINS, MD, MRCS
PETER MACDONALD, MD
R. G. McGOWAN, MD, DPH
A. MURDOCH, MB
A. RUGG-GUNN, MB, FRCS

With regard to (2) I am now satisfied that I can provide my students with the material for getting practical experience in teaching by combining the work of the Teachers' Training School with that of the little school for children and young people which has gradually been developed in connexion with my work. In this school children of all ages are taught how to apply the principles and procedures of my work whilst engaged in the usual school activities, and I am confident that the experience to be gained by combining the work of the students with the work of these children can be of the greatest benefit to all concerned.

With regard to (3) the applications which have come to me

from medical men and from those anxious to make use of the work in the field of education and medicine justify me in believing that the demand for teachers is growing rapidly and that it will probably exceed the supply when we reach the end of the three years' training course (1933). To shew how wide a field is opening out for teachers of my work I may mention that during the past 26 years pupils have come to me, not only from all parts of the British Isles and Ireland, but from several European countries, from Australia, New Zealand, Canada, South Africa, South America, Egypt, India, and the United States of America.* The enquiries from people who have subsequently taken lessons represent, however, a comparatively small proportion of those received from people who are unable to come to London and are anxious to find a teacher of my work nearer their home.

For the benefit of those who have not read my books I must point out that would-be teachers of my work must be trained to put the principles and procedures of its technique into practice in the use of themselves in their daily activities before they attempt to teach others to do likewise. Herein lies the difference between the proposed training and all other forms of training. For students may take courses of training in medicine, physiology, theology, law, philosophy or anything else without the matter of the use of themselves being called into question. But in the training for this teaching a considerable amount of work must be done on the students individually so that they may learn to use themselves satisfactorily, and it is only when they have reached a given standard in the use of themselves that they will be given the opportunity for practical teaching experience.

But, in addition to this individual work, class work will be necessary, and for this part of the work the classes will be confined to five or six students working together with experienced teachers. When students are working together,

*New York, Massachusetts, Connecticut, New Jersey, Pennsylvania, Ohio, Georgia, Alabama, South Carolina, Illinois, Minnesota, Nebraska, California.

however, opportunity will be given to one of the class (a
different one each day) to assume the rôle of guide or adviser
during part of the day's work.

Already two substantial donations have been promised
towards the formation of a Trust Fund for the establishment in
the future of a school in which the teaching posts will be filled
by those who are competent to teach in accordance with the
technique outlined in my books. The Earl of Lytton, Sir
Lynden Macassey and Dr Peter Macdonald have consented to
become Trustees of this Trust Fund, and also Members of a
Society which is being formed to extend in every way the scope
of the work.

22nd July, 1930   F.M.A.

This Appendix is of course now out of date, but reference can
be made to:

      The Secretary
      Alexander Institute
      3B Albert Court
      London S.W.7

INDEX